Palgrave Macmillan Studies in Family and I

Titles include:

Graham Allan, Graham Crow and Sheila Hawker
STEPFAMILIES

Harriet Becher
FAMILY PRACTICES IN SOUTH ASIAN MUSLIM FAMILIES
Parenting in a Multi-Faith Britain

Elisa Rose Birch, Anh T. Le and Paul W. Miller
HOUSEHOLD DIVISIONS OF LABOUR
Teamwork, Gender and Time

Ann Buchanan and Anna Rotkirch
FERTILITY RATES AND POPULATION DECLINE
No Time for Children?

Deborah Chambers
SOCIAL MEDIA AND PERSONAL RELATIONSHIPS
Online Intimacies and Networked Friendship

Robbie Duschinsky and Leon Antonio Rocha (*editors*)
FOUCAULT, THE FAMILY AND POLITICS

Jacqui Gabb
RESEARCHING INTIMACY IN FAMILIES

Stephen Hicks
LESBIAN, GAY AND QUEER PARENTING
Families, Intimacies, Genealogies

Clare Holdsworth
FAMILY AND INTIMATE MOBILITIES

Rachel Hurdley
HOME, MATERIALITY, MEMORY AND BELONGING
Keeping Culture

Peter Jackson (editor)
CHANGING FAMILIES, CHANGING FOOD

Riitta Jallinoja and Eric Widmer (*editors*)
FAMILIES AND KINSHIP IN CONTEMPORARY EUROPE
Rules and Practices of Relatedness

Lynn Jamieson and Roona Simpson (*editors*)
LIVING ALONE
Globalization, Identity and Belonging

Lynn Jamieson, Ruth Lewis and Roona Simpson (*editors*)
RESEARCHING FAMILIES AND RELATIONSHIPS
Reflections on Process

David Morgan
RETHINKING FAMILY PRACTICES

Petra Nordqvist and Carol Smart
RELATIVE STRANGERS: FAMILY LIFE, GENES AND DONOR CONCEPTION

Eriikka Oinonen
FAMILIES IN CONVERGING EUROPE
A Comparison of Forms, Structures and Ideals

Róisín Ryan-Flood
LESBIAN MOTHERHOOD
Gender, Families and Sexual Citizenship

Sally Sales
ADOPTION, FAMILY AND THE PARADOX OF ORIGINS
A Foucauldian History

Tam Sanger
TRANS PEOPLE'S PARTNERSHIPS
Towards an Ethics of Intimacy

Tam Sanger and Yvette Taylor (*editors*)
MAPPING INTIMACIES
Relations, Exchanges, Affects

Elizabeth B. Silva
TECHNOLOGY, CULTURE, FAMILY
Influences on Home Life

Lisa Smyth
THE DEMANDS OF MOTHERHOOD
Agents, Roles and Recognitions

Yvette Taylor
EDUCATIONAL DIVERSITY
The Subject of Difference and Different Subjects

Palgrave Macmillan Studies in Family and Intimate Life
Series Standing Order ISBN 978-0-230-51748-6 hardback
978-0-230-24924-0 paperback
(*outside North America only*)

You can receive future titles in this series as they are published by placing a standing order. Please contact your bookseller or, in case of difficulty, write to us at the address below with your name and address, the title of the series and the ISBN quoted above.

Customer Services Department, Macmillan Distribution Ltd, Houndmills, Basingstoke, Hampshire RG21 6XS, England

---

Relative Strangers: Family Life, Genes and Donor Conception

Petra Nordqvist and Carol Smart

The Morgan Centre, School of Social Sciences, University of Manchester, UK

palgrave
macmillan

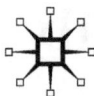

© Petra Nordqvist and Carol Smart 2014

All rights reserved. No reproduction, copy or transmission of this
publication may be made without written permission.

No portion of this publication may be reproduced, copied or transmitted
save with written permission or in accordance with the provisions of the
Copyright, Designs and Patents Act 1988, or under the terms of any licence
permitting limited copying issued by the Copyright Licensing Agency,
Saffron House, 6–10 Kirby Street, London EC1N 8TS.

Any person who does any unauthorized act in relation to this publication
may be liable to criminal prosecution and civil claims for damages.

The authors have asserted their rights to be identified as the authors of this
work in accordance with the Copyright, Designs and Patents Act 1988.

First published 2014 by
PALGRAVE MACMILLAN

Palgrave Macmillan in the UK is an imprint of Macmillan Publishers Limited,
registered in England, company number 785998, of Houndmills, Basingstoke,
Hampshire RG21 6XS.

Palgrave Macmillan in the US is a division of St Martin's Press LLC,
175 Fifth Avenue, New York, NY 10010.

Palgrave Macmillan is the global academic imprint of the above companies
and has companies and representatives throughout the world.

Palgrave® and Macmillan® are registered trademarks in the United States,
the United Kingdom, Europe and other countries.

ISBN 978–1–137–29763–1 hardback
ISBN 978–1–137–29766–2 paperback

This book is printed on paper suitable for recycling and made from fully
managed and sustained forest sources. Logging, pulping and manufacturing
processes are expected to conform to the environmental regulations of the
country of origin.

A catalogue record for this book is available from the British Library.

A catalog record for this book is available from the Library of Congress.

For Iris

Contents

List of Tables and Figures		viii
Series Editors' Preface		ix
Acknowledgements		xi
Introduction		1
1	Proper Families? Cultural Expectations and Donor Conception	11
2	Uncharted Territories: Donor Conception in Personal Life	29
3	Ripples through the Family	48
4	Keeping It Close: Sensitivities and Secrecy	68
5	Opening Up: Disclosure, Information and Family Relationships	87
6	Relating to Donors: Strangers, Boundaries and Tantalising Knowledge	106
7	(Not) One of Us: Genes and Belonging in Everyday Life	125
8	Relative Strangers and the Paradoxes of Genetic Kinship	144
Appendix I: Researching Donor Conception and Family Relationships		166
Appendix II: Index of Participants		173
Appendix III: Glossary of terms		180
Notes		181
Bibliography		183
Index		190

Tables and Figures

Tables

A1 Number of children conceived in the study by gamete donation type (total number of children in the families in the study $N = 111$)   168

A2 Frequency of route to conception (total number of cases $N = 74$)   169

A3 Birth year of participants and donor conceived children in families interviewed ($N = 229$)   169

A4 Ethnic identity of participants (total number of participants $N = 119$)   170

A5 Parent participants' highest level of qualification (total number of parents $N = 78$)   171

Figure

2.1 Visualising dimensions of 'choice'   40

Series Editors' Preface

The remit of the *Palgrave Macmillan Studies in Family and Intimate Life* series is to publish major texts, monographs and edited collections focusing broadly on the sociological exploration of intimate relationships and family organisation. As editors we think such a series is timely. Expectations, commitments and practices have changed significantly in intimate relationships and family life in recent decades. This is very apparent in patterns of family formation and dissolution, demonstrated by trends in cohabitation, marriage and divorce. Changes in household living patterns over the last 20 years have also been marked, with more people living alone, adult children living longer in the parental home, and more 'non-family' households being formed. Furthermore, there have been important shifts in the ways people construct intimate relationships. There are few comfortable certainties about the best ways of being a family man or woman, with once conventional gender roles no longer being widely accepted. The normative connection between sexual relationships and marriage or marriage-like relationships is also less powerful than it once was. Not only is greater sexual experimentation accepted, but it is now accepted at an earlier age. Moreover, heterosexuality is no longer the only mode of sexual relationship given legitimacy. In Britain as elsewhere, gay male and lesbian partnerships are now socially and legally endorsed to a degree hardly imaginable in the mid-twentieth century. Increases in lone-parent families, the rapid growth of different types of step-family, the de-stigmatisation of births outside marriage, and the rise in 'living-apart-together' (LAT) couples all provide further examples of the ways that 'being a couple', 'being a parent' and 'being a family' have diversified in recent years.

The fact that change in family life and intimate relationships has been so pervasive has resulted in renewed research interest from sociologists and other scholars. Increasing amounts of public funding have been directed to family research in recent years, in terms of both individual projects and the creation of family research centres of different hues. This research activity has been accompanied by the publication of some very important and influential books exploring different aspects of shifting family experience, in Britain and elsewhere. The *Palgrave Macmillan Studies in Family and Intimate Life* series hopes to add to this list of influential research-based texts, thereby contributing to existing knowledge and informing current debates. Our main audience consists of academics and advanced students, though we intend that the books in the series will be accessible to a more general readership who wish to understand better the changing nature of contemporary family life and personal relationships.

We see the remit of the series as wide. The concept of 'family and intimate life' is interpreted in a broad fashion. While the focus of the series is clearly sociological, we take family and intimacy as being inclusive rather than exclusive. The series covers a range of topics concerned with family practices and experiences, including, for example, partnership, marriage, parenting, domestic arrangements, kinship, demographic change, intergenerational ties, life course transitions, step-families, gay and lesbian relationships, lone-parent households and non-familial intimate relationships such as friendships. We also wish to foster comparative research, as well as research on under-studied populations. The series includes different forms of book. Most are theoretical or empirical monographs on particular substantive topics, though some may also have a strong methodological focus. In addition, we see edited collections as falling within the series' remit, as well as translations of significant publications in other languages. Finally, we intend the series to have an international appeal, in terms of both topics covered and authorship. Our goal is for the series to provide a forum for family sociologists conducting research in various societies, and not solely in Britain.

Graham Allan, Lynn Jamieson and David Morgan

Acknowledgements

We would like to thank the Economic and Social Research Council (ESRC) for generously funding the research on which this book is based. Details of the project, which was called 'Relative Strangers: Negotiating Non-Genetic Kinship in the Context of Assisted Conception', can be found on the ESRC website (ESRC reference: RES-062-23-2810). In particular we wish to mention Michelle Dodson of the ESRC, who offered us guidance in the last stages of the project. We are also grateful to the trustees of the Mass Observation Archive at the University of Sussex for permission to reproduce Mass Observation material in Chapter 1. The project was based at the Morgan Centre for the Study of Relationships and Personal Life at the University of Manchester and we thank all our colleagues there for their support and encouragement during the course of the research. We are grateful to Jennifer Mason, Sue Heath, Vanessa May, Brian Heaphy, Paul Simpson, Gemma Edwards and Wendy Bottero for all their stimulating comments and contributions over the years. Our particular thanks go to Victoria Higham, Hazel Burke, Lisa Jenkins and Louise McMahon, who, in their different ways, kept the project organised and on track for three years. We are also immensely grateful to the Donor Conception Network, who have been keenly interested in our research and were also so helpful in assisting us to recruit many heterosexual couples for our study. Local Lesbian Mums groups were also invaluable in helping us to recruit lesbian couples and we list other organisations who helped us along our way in Appendix I. Finally our thanks go to all the parents and grandparents who participated in our project, without whom none of this would have been possible.

Introduction

Victoria and Jeffrey lived with their children in a small rural village in the South of England. As they were a heterosexual married couple with two small children, their family may have looked quite typical from the outside. However, there was an aspect to their story which was unusual, and this meant that they faced unusual kinds of ethical and social dilemmas in their family life. To become parents, they had gone through three years of very intensive in vitro fertilisation (IVF) treatments which failed because the quality of Jeffrey's sperm was too poor. So they made the decision to use donor sperm. This meant that they had to face the dilemma of whether to tell their children about the donor and their genetic background. While Jeffrey and Victoria were going through counselling at the fertility clinic, they decided that, if they were successful, they would tell their child about his or her origins. At the time of the interview they had two children, the elder a four-year-old girl. Victoria had been very committed to explaining all about sperm donation to her daughter from a very early age and they had followed advice on how to do this with the help of dedicated self-help books and also using agreed terminology (e.g. the sperm donor was always called Mr Donor). But what Victoria was not prepared for was the fact that, after she had told her daughter about her conception, the child would then make this information available to everybody in the very small village in which they lived. Victoria told us the following story:

> We were just sitting in the room waiting for the vet to come in [and] the waiting room was right next to us, filled with people with

their dogs and everything. And [my daughter] just suddenly said, 'Oh, mummy, you really wanted a baby, didn't you?' And I said, (laughter), 'Yes.' And then she said, 'And daddy's sperm didn't work,' in this clear little singsong voice. 'So we asked Mr Donor and he...' It sounded really sort of dirty and horrid, I don't know. She said, 'And we got it from another man,' she didn't even say a kind man I don't think. But obviously I just had to say, 'That's right, darling, well done, you've remembered it really well' and [I was] feeling incredibly embarrassed. And that's the first time I've had to be, sort of, just be exposed, I suppose. Because I'm really, you know, it's very important to me that people understand it, so when I tell I can actually explain it to people. But I couldn't sort of then go into the waiting room and say, 'Right, I need to explain why.' You know, because of course you can't. So it was quite embarrassing, but it's going to happen again, you know.

This is a very typical story of the sort of dilemma that parents of donor conceived children face. If they want to be open with their children they discover very quickly that sensitive information about their own private problems of infertility and their chosen method of conception becomes public property. In the story above it is revealed that it is impossible to tell children about their conception and then ask them to keep it secret from strangers. Victoria's discomfort is obvious and understandable. She says she would prefer to explain things to people in her own way so that they would not misconstrue what had gone on, but she realises that she had lost control of the information. She was particularly unhappy that her daughter had not referred to Mr Donor as a *kind* man, perhaps because she feared that people might think she had gone off for a one-night stand with a stranger. Her story not only reveals the kinds of dilemmas that parents in this situation have to face but it also reminds us of how vulnerable they can feel in a community which takes for granted that children are the genetic offspring of their parents and where infertility may still be stigmatised.

This story reveals the way in which the parents of donor conceived children face all kinds of unexpected situations not typically encountered in everyday family life. Such parents also have to solve unanticipated dilemmas, such as whether it is better to find a donor from within the wider family rather than from a pool of strangers or whether donors should be involved in some way in the lives of the children they help to generate. They have to decide whether to go abroad to find gametes because waiting times can be too long in the UK, and then they have to decide whether to go to a country where there is complete donor anonymity or whether to go to one which will allow their hoped-for child to find their donor when they are older. At present these sorts of issues are real challenges to parents and sometimes even an awful burden. We found that when would-be parents are going through the process of trying to conceive against the odds, they are focused on achieving a pregnancy rather than working out exactly what they will do about hypothetical problems that may arise some years later. Although sketching out certain principles in advance (for example whether to tell children of their conception or whether to choose a known or unknown donor) is important, circumstances can also change dramatically, making early decisions inappropriate. Alternatively, would-be parents may find that they cannot actually engineer the circumstances of conception as they may have hoped. In the UK prospective parents who use licensed clinics to access donor conception are provided with counselling, but some couples may go abroad to clinics where there is little or no counselling, and some lesbian couples may use more informal methods of sperm donation and so do not attend a clinic at all. This means that parents embarking on donor conceived parenthood may have little grasp of the issues they are likely to face, and even those who feel well prepared may find that the reality is more challenging than they anticipate.

It is true that sperm donation (which used to be called artificial insemination by donor) is not a new practice, but until relatively recently it was a secret affair and we have little knowledge of how couples in the past in the UK managed the issues that this form of conception must have generated for them. The growth in the numbers of children born through these methods (more than 35,000 in the UK since 1991) combined with changing policies on matters of anonymity of donors and the extension of assisted reproduction methods to single women and lesbians means that the challenges that face parents who conceive children in this way are becoming more topical and less private. However people may come to the difficult decision to use donor gametes, the parents of donor conceived children are entering into a new way of doing family life.

Whether the parents are a heterosexual couple who have unexpectedly discovered that one or both of them have an infertility problem which cannot be solved through standard IVF treatments or intracytoplasmic sperm injection (ICSI), or a lesbian couple, or a single woman who has decided that the only way to have a child is to opt for sperm donation, it introduces new and unprecedented questions for parents and families.

In this book we explore how both heterosexual and lesbian couples and their families are dealing with these modern challenges. We draw on in-depth interviews with 22 heterosexual couples and 22 lesbian couples recruited across England and Wales. We also draw on interviews with 30 grandparents of donor conceived children, 15 of whom had a heterosexual son or daughter and 15 whose daughters were lesbian. We were specifically investigating the situation of couples and their wider families, because within the framework of the study we were exploring the particular issue of how families experience having both genetic and non-genetic connections within families created through donor conception (we explain in more detail how we conducted the study in Appendix I).

In many ways the parents we interviewed for the study were pioneers, and their experiences throw into sharp relief cultural beliefs about family life as well as the consequences of doing family slightly differently. These parents were also unwitting pioneers because by sheer chance they found themselves opting for donor conception precisely at a time when public policy on issues of donor anonymity was changing but had not settled into a generally accepted pattern. From a broader perspective we can also see that they embarked on the process just as popular discourses on the importance of genes and genetic connections reached a kind of zenith. Twenty years earlier they might have found themselves in a cultural context in which the term 'genes' was rarely used and the supposed significance of genetic connection was far more muted than it is today. But British society (along with many others in the West) has undergone a kind of 'geneticisation' of the popular imagination, such that now genes are increasingly believed to be of overwhelming significance in every aspect of life. In such a context not being the genetic parent of one's child might assume a greater significance than formerly and, almost certainly, the idea that it is important to know precisely who one's genetic progenitors are has really gripped the popular consciousness.

The modern experiences which we discuss are of course specific and local to the families who took part in our study. But they are also part of significant social and cultural changes in reproductive practices and family life in Britain and internationally, made possible through developments in medicine in the field of reproductive technologies. The birth of the first IVF baby, Louise Brown, in 1978 in Britain marked the beginning of an expansion of a medicalised infertility industry (Mamo, 2007), and with that the development of a plethora of technologies that assist conception. These medical advances have led to new and unprecedented possibilities in human reproduction. Technologies now enable, for example, ICSI (a technology that allows the insertion of a single sperm into a human egg in vitro) and notable new possibilities such as egg and embryo donation. Reproductive technologies have not only become more sophisticated over the years, but have also become much more commonplace so that people can turn to these technologies more readily when faced with problems of infertility. Data from the Human Fertilisation and Embryology Authority (HFEA), brought into being by the 1990 Human Fertilisation and Embryology Act, shows that between 1992 (when the register started) and 2007, the number of women treated with IVF and ICSI increased by over 250 per cent (HFEA, 2013a). As these technologies have become more widespread, they have also developed a strong international dimension. People who access reproductive care today do not only do so in their own countries, but also turn to clinics abroad, a phenomenon that has become known as cross-border reproductive care or CBRC (Culley *et al.*, 2011). It is difficult to estimate how many couples have sought CBRC so far, but according to Shenfield *et al.* (2010), who analysed data gathered from 46 clinics in Belgium, the Czech Republic, Denmark, Switzerland, Slovenia and Spain, there could be 24,000–30,000 cycles of cross-border treatment (involving 11,000–14,000 patients) taking place in Europe alone every year.

Alongside the developments in medical technologies, the perception of how society should manage these developments in family life has also changed and this has led to new policies and regulations. One particularly important debate in recent years, in the UK and internationally, has been whether the donor conceived child should have access to the identity of the donor. In the UK, this debate culminated in a shift from donor anonymity to donor identity release in

April 2005. Since then, the UK has operated an identity release system so that any child conceived after this date can seek identifying information about their donor at the age of 18. However, this development covers only licensed donor conception in the UK, and given that children are conceived through donation in other ways too, not all donor conceived children born today have the same access to donor information. For example, children born through informal arrangements where couples and donors make their own decisions about contact and information sharing may have more access to information compared with children conceived in licensed clinics, or none at all. Children conceived by donation abroad are also likely to have a different level of access to information as different countries operate different policies on identity release. There are also the children (many of whom are now adults) conceived using licensed UK clinics before April 2005, who have no formal access to information about their donor. However, for a child to access any of this information, he or she must have been told about being donor conceived in the first place. Because of this range of practices around donor identity release/anonymity, the circumstances of individual donor conceived children, and their families, vary considerably.

This diversity in terms of children's access to donor information is part of a larger picture of family diversity that characterises the families that we interviewed for our study. The couples in our study used egg, sperm and embryo donation and, as we shall explore in the chapters that follow, these different pathways afforded couples different experiences of reproductive donation. As we also go on to explain, the sexuality of the couple was often decisive in how they experienced becoming a family. Many of the families we spoke to had accessed treatment in a UK reproductive health centre, but others had found that the waiting lists and costs associated with British treatment were insurmountable and that they could access faster and cheaper treatment abroad. Still other couples, specifically the lesbians in this study, chose to circumvent medical reproductive care altogether and conceived in informal arrangements with sperm donors. Until 2007, it was also possible to use Internet companies to have fresh donor sperm delivered to your door in the UK (a commercial practice which has since been criminalised),[1] and so there are also families with young children conceived outside the clinic context but through a commercial route. Some families had children who could access information about their donor; others did not. In some families the donors were known to the child and the parents; others had never met their donor. This diversity is an integral part of what we call 'families by donation' and in the following chapters we explore both commonalities and differences among them.

In Chapter 1 we start by asking the question of what a 'proper' family looks like. Because the shape and size of families in the UK has changed so much over the last century there has been an endless culture war over which sorts of family are 'real' families. Donor conceived families are the most recent of the new families and they are facing sensitive issues about whether they can fit in and look just like other families or whether they should embrace their difference while still insisting that they are perfectly proper families. This chapter raises in outline some of the dilemmas that the parents and grandparents in our study face while also mapping out the approach we take to understanding contemporary family life. Chapters 2 to 7 are based on the empirical material we collected in carrying out the study. The first of these empirical chapters is titled 'Uncharted Territories' because we explore the journeys that the would-be parents in our study went on to achieve parenthood against the odds. Because the odds facing heterosexual and lesbian couples are not exactly the same, in this chapter we discuss their experiences separately. The heterosexual couples have to face questions about their masculinity (for infertile men) and their womanhood (for infertile women) and the accounts they provide of dealing with these fundamental problems, as well as deciding whether or not to proceed with donor conception, set the scene for later chapters which explore what happens once the baby has arrived. For the lesbian couples our interviews reveal that they face a different set of dilemmas such as whether to go to a licensed clinic or whether to ask a male friend to help, or whether to parent as a couple or to involve their donor in the life of the child. For these couples, unlike the heterosexual couples, the birth of a child does not mean that they can adopt the mantle of a traditional family because they cannot disguise the fact that they have a donor conceived child. But the challenges they face are just as ethically taxing. Chapter 3 focuses on how the advent of a donor conceived child sends ripples through the wider family. Often it is forgotten that donor conception does not only involve the would-be parents and their hoped-for child, and we found that mothers, fathers, mothers-in-law, fathers-in-law, brothers, sisters, cousins and so on may all become involved or have a stake in the new family. We discovered that the older generation could be central in providing support during infertility treatment, especially for heterosexual women, but for lesbian couples wider families could sometimes be less welcoming of the news of a child. In this chapter we begin to map out how important the interactions between family members are once a child is born and we point to the ways in which both lesbian and heterosexual couples are firmly situated in these webs of relationships. Chapters 4 and 5 address the really difficult issues that parents and grandparents face about being open or secretive about their families by donation. In the context of lesbian donation we found that decisions about openness and secrecy in families were as much about the issue of the couples' sexuality as the issue of donor conception. Some people felt very private about a child being born by donation, and wanted to keep the information to themselves as much as possible. We found that parents could be committed to telling their children about their donor origins, but otherwise be quite unwilling to share the information. But we also discovered that family members could play a decisive role in information sharing. We found that sensitivities started to develop in family networks because of this desire to keep some things hidden from public view. In Chapter 5, 'Opening Up: Negotiating Disclosure', we go on to explore the accounts of families who want to share information more widely. We look specifically at how parents negotiated being open because we found that although parents might be committed to sharing information with their child, as well as with others, many found that opening up, and establishing open lines of communication in families, was far from straightforward. Parents encountered significant challenges when explaining donor conception both to their children and to members of their families, and in this chapter we start to map the terrain that parents who sought openness are negotiating in the absence of an established narrative about donation.

One of the central reasons why donor conception gives rise to so many questions in families of donor conceived children is the unusual mapping of genetic connections, within the family as well as across its boundaries to the donor. In Chapters 6 to 8 we explore the meaning of connectedness and belonging in these families, and specifically the meaning of genetic connections. We start in

Chapter 6 by exploring the connection to the donor, and how families relate to him or her. The majority of the couples in our study had conceived using an unknown gamete donor, so the donor was someone they had never met in person. It might be assumed that couples who had no social relationship with the donor would not necessarily dwell on their connection with him or her after the moment of conception, but we found that they continued to relate to the donor and that this connection introduced unusual questions into their lives as the child grew up. A proportion of the families had also used a known donor (for example a friend or someone from the wider family) and these arrangements also initiated unanticipated questions into the lives of these families. One dimension that we explore in this chapter was that the donation did not only connect the child to the donor, but also to his or her wider genetic kin and so, potentially, the child was connected to a whole set of 'relative strangers': siblings, grandparents, aunts, uncles, cousins and so on. This chapter explores how the families managed and perceived this potential proliferation of 'donor kinship'. In Chapter 7, '(Not) One of Us: Genes and Belonging in Family Life', we go on to explore how the families perceived the existence of genetic links *within* their own family. Many found the idea of using donor conception deeply challenging because donor eggs, sperm or embryos introduced questions about whether and how the parents and grandparents could claim the donor conceived child 'as their own' and whether the child was 'a child of the family'. In this chapter we explore how the concepts of genes and blood gave rise to a range of feelings in these families, because the donor conceived child was simultaneously perceived as a child who belonged, while also being different.

In the final chapter, 'Relative Strangers and the Paradoxes of Genetic Kinship', we focus attention on the ways in which ideas about genes and genetic connectedness have come to be so central to our donor conceived families and also to the broader society. We note how popular terminology has shifted from references to blood as a way of connecting kin to ideas about genes. There are many important scientific developments in what is often called the new biology, and media coverage of the links between genes, health and even behaviour is often alarmist and misguided. So here we consider how these kinds of messages are received and what the new emphasis on genetic connections might mean for the ways in which families think about kinship and connectedness. We found that a very complex picture emerged but in the main it did not support the idea that kinship is simply all about genetics.

Assisted donor conception is a field that is constantly developing, and the terminology is often complex and cumbersome. We have found the term 'reproductive donation' (Richards, Pennings and Appleby, 2012) useful, because although perhaps formal, it works as a shorthand to describe the practice involved. In the following chapters we will at times refer to 'heterosexual donation' and 'lesbian donation', to describe the family form of which our participants speak. In order not to encumber the reader with too much description of the participants' individual family situation, we refer to them by numbers, and the reader can cross-reference to the index of participants at the back of the book. We have also included a glossary explaining complex terminology in the field.

1
Proper Families? Cultural Expectations and Donor Conception

Judges are asked to rule over child who has 'three parents'
(*The Times* Tuesday February 7, 2012)

Such headlines in the UK are now far from rare. For example, in February 2013 alone *The Guardian* had two similar articles; one was headed 'Who's my sperm donor father?' (February 23, 2013) and the other stated 'Our kids have two mums' (February 16, 2013). Similar headlines would have been unthinkable 50 or even 20 years ago and perhaps what is most surprising about such media coverage is that, although the tabloid press might take a more 'shock/horror' approach to such stories, in the main they are presented as news stories which just reflect the changing shape and structure of contemporary family life. These stories challenge, and ultimately may start to redefine, taken-for-granted assumptions about motherhood, fatherhood and what constitutes a 'real' or 'proper' family. So the question we open this chapter with is 'What constitutes a proper family?'

The dominant cultural narrative about family life is still largely based on the idea of a married heterosexual couple who live together with their 'own' genetic children (usually just two of them). Even though this idealised model has never fully represented the diversity of family life in the UK, until recently it has been a powerful image which not only seemed to represent the actuality of lived experience but also became the moral standard of what families *should* be like (Gillis, 1996). Thus people who did not fit exactly within this model were often seen as undesirable or as harming their children (e.g. Rights of Women, 1984). The idea that all proper families must consist of married heterosexual parents and their two children reached a pinnacle in the 1950s and 1960s when marriage rates soared to their highest in recorded times (Allan and Crow, 2001; Lewis, 2001; McRae, 2004) and when any form of deviation from this ideal led to ostracism and sometimes even legal intervention (Keating, 2009; Sales, 2012). These marginalised, even stigmatised families might have included families with illegitimate children, single-parent families, adoptive families, mixed-race or mixed-religion families, same-sex families, unmarried families, small families, large families and so on.

Given the strength of the ideal or 'proper' form of family in the popular imagination until quite recently,[1] it is hardly surprising that, even now, new family forms materialising out of changing social, legal and cultural conditions can cause worry, alarm and sometimes dismay in some quarters. Hence for many years the growth in divorce and the rise of lone-parent families, particularly in the 1980s in the UK, was met with distress and condemnation in almost equal measure (Morgan, 1995; 2000).The first 'test-tube baby' (Louise Brown) was welcomed as a miracle but also as an indicator that families might start working against nature to produce 'designer' babies. Even the practice of adopting children in the early twentieth century was seen as a way of damaging the proper family because unmarried mothers could too 'easily' rid themselves of the burden of their sins and thus serve to condone sex outside marriage.

Adverse reactions to novel or changing family forms are therefore far from new and families formed through assisted reproductive methods, especially those using donated gametes, are now under this kind of fretful scrutiny. Some families find themselves under particularly close examination because their private lives come to public notice when they have gone to court to solve a particular family conflict or problem. Such cases give rise to the kinds of headlines in newspapers that we feature at the start of this chapter.

So in this chapter we first want to explore what it means when issues of donor conception enter into a semi-public, legal forum because this type of event provides insights into how society responds to these new family forms. Focusing on one case will allow us to discuss cultural ideas about what constitutes 'proper' families and the importance, or otherwise, of blood connections within such families. We will then consider child adoption because this practice is frequently seen as analogous to donor conception and it is often argued that the principles governing adoption should apply to donor conception. We will explore how the practice of adoption was also originally seen as undesirable, how it became shrouded in secrecy and how this has given way to open adoption where a child knows about their birth parents. Following this, the question of personal identity will be explored because a core contemporary concern around donor conception is the idea that the child who is detached in some way from genetic kin (formerly blood kin) will suffer a loss of identity (Marshall, 2012). We suggest, however, that rather than a focus on the idea of identity, a broader notion of 'belonging' is a more appropriate way to understand these new families. Finally we focus on the new narratives of family life that are emerging and how they bring with them new frameworks for understanding what families 'should' be like. In our conclusion we will outline the broad theoretical stance that informs this study and which is referred to as the relational approach.

The case of *ML & AR v RW-B & SW-B [2011]*[2]

Court cases can be seen to occupy an important symbolic place in the process of forming public opinion about family change. The details of cases involving donor conception (e.g. a child having two mothers or the rights of sperm donors to obtain legal privileges in relation to genetic children) inform a wider public of these otherwise private practices. They also put such events into context and at the same time can be very suggestive of whether these new family practices are desirable or not. The more the general public reads about these cases, the more they become aware of different forms of family life, whether they ultimately approve of them or not.

The legal case we focus on involved a lesbian couple who we refer to here as Rosie and Sally and a gay couple we refer to as Mark and Andrew. These are not their real names because although the details of their lives are in the public domain, they still have the right to anonymity. The facts of their dispute are not particularly unusual and the issues at stake are ones that face many gay and lesbian couples when they decide to have children through informal sperm donation. That is to say, they did not go through a licensed clinic to receive donor sperm because, if they had, the donor would have given up his rights to claim legal paternity of the children born from his gametes. Although this dispute may seem to be relevant only to same-sex couples using informal methods for conceiving children, the principles in play have a much wider currency. This is because there are important social values and ethical questions at stake. For example, in any situation where a gamete donor is already known to a recipient (e.g. a cousin who donates her eggs) there are commanding questions about how much of a role a donor should have in the life of a child they have helped to create (and we explore some of these questions further in Chapter 6). So the case of Rosie and Sally is not just about same-sex parents, it is also about how to establish who a parent is, and also whether 'degrees of parenthood' can be apportioned, such that a donor might have a small 'share' in parenting while the birth mother (in egg donation) or the non-genetic father (in sperm donation) might have a larger share. This case, and others like it, raises the question of whether parenthood can be envisaged as a kind of 'parenthood pie chart' which is no longer comprised of two equal parts taken by two genetic parents, but of several different adults who each have a different-sized slice of the pie or a different role to play.

The story

Rosie and Sally decided they wanted children together so they advertised for a gay man who would be willing to donate sperm. Mark volunteered. He was in a long-term relationship with Andrew. The couples met and decided to proceed with the plan with a general understanding that Mark would be a father figure to any subsequent child who was born. A daughter, who we call Paula, was born in 2001 and a second daughter, who we call Lilly, was born in 2005. Mark was the genetic father of both Paula and Lilly, and Rosie was the genetic and birth mother of both of the girls. Sally had parental responsibility for both girls arising from her civil partnership with Rosie. Mark and Andrew saw a lot of Paula and Lilly, taking them on holiday and having them to stay with them. During this period of the couples' relationship it is possible to envisage the arrangement of the 'parenthood pie chart' with Rosie and Sally both having the larger slices, but with Mark having a growing slice and Andrew sharing in Mark's portion. The girls referred to Mark as 'Daddy' at this time. However, in 2008 the relationship between the couples deteriorated rapidly; it seems that Mark and Andrew moved house to be closer to the girls and they began to want to have more time with them and to have a greater say in decision-making. The relationship between Mark (as a genetic progenitor) and Sally (as a non-genetic parent) became particularly strained. Conflict erupted and the couples went to court because Rosie and Sally wanted to reduce the amount of contact their daughters had with Mark and Andrew, but Mark wanted to be recognised as the legal father of the girls, and not only demanded more contact, but also made a claim for residence. This meant that he wanted the children to be removed from Rosie and Sally in order to come to live with him and Andrew. By reference to the 'parenthood pie chart' again, we can see that Mark saw himself in the same position as that of a divorced heterosexual father who could assume he was entitled to 50 per cent of the metaphorical pie, leaving the other 50 per cent (or possibly a bit less) to Rosie. Rosie and Sally were, however, only willing to concede about 10 per cent of the pie to Mark and Andrew.

The problem with this pie chart analogy, of course, is that it allows one to forget that these were real people arguing over actual children who were caught in the middle of stressful legal proceedings for at least three years. Paula, the elder daughter, was ten years old at the time of the final court hearing and by then she was refusing to see Mark at all even though Mark was insistent upon it. The contact facilitator reported to the court that Paula had said the following:

> P told me that she wished she could move away, far away from all this conflict, all this horrible stuff. She told me that she cries at school in the toilets and her friend looks after her when she is upset, which is a lot. P said that she does not feel as if M is a father to her. She has two mothers. That is her family and she is happy with that. She liked M and A and likes seeing them too, but she did not think of them as her family because she has family. It is the mothers and her younger sister. She cannot just pretend that M is her father in order to make him happy.
>
> (*ML & AR v RW-B & SW-B [2011]* para 2)

The ingredients of this case are exactly the same components that are to be found wherever donor conception results in the birth of a child. By this we mean that there are always more than two adults involved in donor conception and this can give rise to new dimensions of conflict when relationships break down. As a society we have become familiar with court cases dealing with divorced heterosexual parents who cannot agree about who a child should live with or how much contact a parent should have (Smart and Neale, 1999; Smart *et al.*, 2001). We are less familiar with instances where there are three or even four people claiming parental rights. Although it is now quite accepted that a child can be raised by two mothers, or that a heterosexual couple can use gamete donation to have a child, uncertainty still hovers over the status of the donor and the donor's family, and also whether the child born of donor conception should have some kind of legally recognised relationship or kinship with the donor and his or her other kin.

When sperm donation started to become an accepted method of dealing with male infertility in the UK around the time of the Second World War, so threatening was the figure of the donor that doctors and parents colluded in order to write him out of history and basically allowed the husband to assume legal parenthood of any child born from the method (Daniels and Haimes, 1998; Richards *et al.*, 2012). The potential claim of the genetic donor was simply defused in order that the receiving parents could feel secure in their status as 'real' parents and so that they could present themselves to a potentially hostile society as a proper family. The case of Rosie and Sally some 70 years later contains echoes of this same scenario where the looming donor can make claims to a child, even though the child is happy with the family they already have. The facts in our modern case are not quite as straightforward as this because Mark, the sperm donor, was also the acknowledged father figure (or daddy), but it was his genetic connection with the girls that allowed him to go to court and this shows how socially and legally powerful genetic relatedness can be. While, in the 1950s, it was heterosexual couples who feared that the sperm donor could undermine their family, in the 2010s it is lesbian couples who experience this fear. It may also be an apprehension shared by any parent of a donor conceived child where the donor is known to them and their family.

So in some circumstances genetic connections give rise to legal standing (the right to make a claim) and possibly legal status (having one's claim recognised). But not all genetic connections do this.

A brother cannot, for example, make claims on a sister who would be legally recognised and grandparents can only rarely make legal claims in relation to grandchildren. It is genetic connection through sperm, eggs or embryos that carries this particular social, legal and cultural power. The legal conflict between Rosie, Sally, Mark and Andrew reveals that there is no automatic assumption that donor conceived families will be treated in the same way as families comprising parents with their own genetic children. In such circumstances it is not surprising that the former are anxious still to be seen as 'proper' families (Nordqvist, 2012a).

The question that flows from this realisation is whether it is a good thing that as a society we are moving towards the recognition that a child can have multiple parents, each of whom has a 'stake' in the child and who brings to the child a wider kinship network, or whether it would be a better thing if social and legal values preserved the idea that there really should only ever be two acknowledged parents because this is what is expected of 'proper' families (Wallbank, 2002). There are no easy answers to this question. As we discuss in the chapters that follow, the parents of donor conceived children often feel very vulnerable and want to benefit from the perceived protections conferred on genetically related or 'proper' families. Yet at the same time many lesbian parents (like Rosie and Sally) actively seek out an involved father figure for their children and many heterosexual parents propose to tell their children about their donors. Some parents are therefore trying to reshape parenthood away from the familiar twosome model towards a different combination of adults, while insisting that this too is a proper family. Putting it simply, there is an ongoing contest between the traditional ideals of a 'proper' family and more emergent aspirations that proper families can take many different shapes.

Learning from adoption?

There are striking parallels between the story of adoption in the UK and the development of policy and principles governing donor conception. But the stories are not identical and it would be inappropriate to assume that donor conception should simply be forced into the tracks left behind from the arduous journey taken by adoption (Haimes, 1988). At all times it is vital to remember how much society has changed over the last century and to realise that some of the experiences that were so influential in the development of adoption policies may hold little relevance for donor conception.

In England and Wales we can readily identify when the practice of legal adoption as we recognise it today began. The Adoption Act of 1926 created a system in which parents wishing to relinquish their child or children could place them for adoption. Suitable adoptive parents would then be found and there would follow a legal process whereby birth parents gave up their legal parental rights, which were transferred to the adoptive parents. Once an adoption order was made birth parents could not change their minds and they could never have the child returned to them. They were absolved of any financial or legal responsibilities for the child and in effect were no longer regarded as kin. The adoptive parents became the sole parents and, if the child had been born illegitimate, the adoption order removed the legal stigma and the child became the legitimate child of his or her new parents. This policy firmly shaped the 'proper' adoptive family of the 1930s and subsequent decades into the increasingly dominant two-parent model. It is not clear how extensive this model was before 1926, however. As Jenny Keating (2009) and Sally Sales (2012) have shown, adoption did exist before 1926 but it was not regulated and it was referred to later as informal adoption to distinguish it from the state-regulated, legal variety. The most important difference between adoption pre- and post-1926 was that before the Adoption Act, birth parents could take their children back. They retained their kinship with their children and were expected to contribute financially towards the children's upkeep. This latter policy was to prevent parents from lodging their children with adoptive parents while they were costly (and unproductive) infants only to claim them back as soon as they could earn a living. There is also evidence of informal intra-family adoption; for instance, an illegitimate child might be sent to be raised by an aunt and uncle, or a grandmother might simply assume the maternal role for an illegitimate child born to her daughter. In these latter cases children often never knew that the person they thought was their older sister was in fact their mother.[3] The three extracts below, from the Mass Observation Archive at Sussex University, were written in 2000 and show how the practice of informal and intra-family adoptions still exists in living memory:

I know one of the aunts had an unexpected baby but the little one just got tacked on to the large family of another aunt.

(P425 Female, aged 62, ex-nurse, married)

I understand that [my aunt] pretty well dumped the child on her own mother. This cousin was pushed from pillar to post and lived with me and my parents for a short while. All three offspring went to university, held commissions in the services and are solid and respectable citizens to my knowledge. The illegitimate child (who is more or less an age with me) seems to have done well enough.

(B2238 Male, aged 76, retired clergyman, married)

One thing that has always fascinated me about my own and my wife's fairly recent ancestors is the level of pre-marital sex that clearly occurred, if you compare birth and marriage certificates, and the casual way children were treated. It seems to me that the early part of the Century, despite the prudishness associated with it, was full of illicit relations and illegal adoptions....My grandfather once told me about Doris. She was child number 10 or 11 and my grandmother couldn't cope. Doris was given to a nearby neighbour and brought up by them not knowing who her real parents were until she was going to get married and needed her father to sign an agreement. Only then did she discover, in a state of complete shock, that 'uncle' Bill was her dad.

(P2759 Male, 50, married, director, S. Wales)

There is no way of knowing how many of these informal adoptions there were; nor can we ascertain whether they were kept secret or were more like open secrets that families lived with. But it is quite clear that such practices were acceptable and even essential (when illegitimacy and lone motherhood were so reviled) giving rise to situations where immediate kin could be spread across different households and not kept within the confines of the two-parent, nuclear family. The rise of state-regulated adoption gradually changed these practices and, combined with the lessening of the stigma of lone motherhood, the abolition of the legal status of illegitimacy and the rise of birth control, it meant that by the end of the twentieth century the whole practice of adoption had been transformed. The era of mother-and-baby homes, where young pregnant women were sent to have their babies in clandestine surroundings and to put them up secretly for adoption (Spensky, 1992), occupied a relatively short period of time in the longer history of adoption in England. In the 1950s and 1960s young women often reluctantly relinquished their babies and, once they had done so, they were never allowed to see them again. Moreover, during those decades there was a surplus of babies available for adoption and so adoptive parents were at a premium and their desire to be unencumbered by the potential ghost of the birth mother influenced adoption societies to promote adoption policies which de-kinned birth parents from their children (Sales, 2012).

This policy of secret adoptions (where children were not told they were adopted and where birth parents were completely cut off) fell into disrepute by the end of the century. There were a number of factors involved in this changed mindset. The numbers of babies available for adoption fell and children who became available for adoption were increasingly those who had been removed from their families by the local authority because of neglect or mistreatment. These were older children who often had problems but who also knew who their birth parents were. Sometimes they had spent periods of time in a children's home or in foster care and so their adoptive parents were not in a position to 'pretend' to be their birth parents. As Jane Lewis (2004) has shown, the other important change to adoption across the second half of the twentieth century was that it ceased to be a way of providing babies for childless couples and instead became a part of the state's child care system. Adoption became a solution for children, not for parents who did not want another child, nor for would-be parents who wanted a child to complete their family. Most significantly, in the UK the state retains an overarching role in the practice of adoption and, through the offices of local authority social workers, has the power to decide who is deemed to be a suitable adoptive parent.

The history of assisted reproduction maps onto some of these historical trends imperfectly. While we know little about sperm donation before the Second World War, in the post-war decades it seems that some doctors were willing to provide what was known as artificial insemination by donor to childless married couples (Richards, 2006). The practice was veiled, not because it was illegal but because it was seen as so shameful. It is also clear that doctors at that time, and even until the turn of the twentieth century, were advising couples not to tell their children about the unusual nature of their conception. English family law worked on the presumption that children born to a married woman were the legitimate offspring of her husband and so there was no requirement for any kind of legal steps to be taken for these infertile husbands to become legal parents. As a consequence there are no records at all of how many children may have been born from this type of assisted conception. The significant parallel with adoption policy during the 1950s and 1960s resides in the fact that both adoption societies and infertility doctors were advising parents to keep secret the detail that their children were not (fully) their genetic offspring. So in both spheres policy leant heavily towards preserving the image of the 'proper' family as one including only two parents and their own genetic children.

Thereafter policies began to diverge considerably. While policy on adoption began to move (back) towards greater openness about parenthood, assisted reproduction continued to be a private and sometimes secret matter. It is important to understand that from the 1970s onwards most technical developments in assisted reproduction were designed to help childless couples to conceive a child with their own gametes. Methods such as in vitro fertilisation (IVF), gamete intra-fallopian transfer (GIFT) or intra-cytoplasmic sperm injection (ICSI) have all been pursued to find ways to ensure that heterosexual couples could conceive in this way. Sperm donation remained important, but the Holy Grail of treatment was to perfect methods which did not need to introduce gametes from a third party. This means that assisted reproduction in general progressed according to very different kinds of aims and values compared with adoption. With assisted reproduction there might never be a baby, while with adoption there was a child already in existence. Assisted reproduction was a service for childless couples (and latterly single women and same-sex couples) but adoption was a service for children in need. The introduction of embryo and egg donation/sharing was also, in many ways, an offshoot of the social and financial organisation of assisted reproduction rather than a goal in itself. Technologies of safely freezing and preserving embryos and eggs are relatively recent, and they developed as a way of avoiding the waste of eggs caused by super-ovulatory drugs given to women undergoing IVF. Once doctors abandoned the early practice of introducing six or seven embryos back into the womb (often giving rise to multiple births and babies with severe disabilities) they needed a way to preserve the unused eggs and embryos for possible future use, or even for the use of other women. This in turn gave rise to the now common practice of egg sharing between women undergoing treatments, which not only ensures that surplus eggs are utilised but also helps to reduce the financial cost of services which are not always available on the UK National Health Service (NHS).

Tracing this history reveals very different motivations embedded within the development of donor conception, compared with the motivation of child-saving which epitomises recent policies on adoption. However, these two parallel tracks are beginning to move closer together again. The state, through the Human Fertilisation and Embryology Authority (HFEA) and the regulation of infertility clinics, has become more closely involved with assisted reproduction and has even legislated in the past for the kinds of potential parents it prefers. This originally meant that only heterosexual couples were entitled to reproductive health care treatment, but this gradually relaxed until the stage was reached where (as with adoption) single women and lesbian couples could access treatment. The state has also abolished anonymous gamete donation in all UK licensed infertility clinics and from April 2005 all children conceived in this way are entitled to receive identifying information about their donors when they reach the age of 18. The most significant potential policy overlap between donor conception and adoption now is precisely in this area of creating and/or sustaining links with genetic parents. It is, for example, possible to argue that just as adoption policy has realised the importance for children of knowing their birth parents, so donor conception policy should step into line and acknowledge the importance of children knowing their genetic forebears (Turkmendag, 2012). However, there is a significant slippage in terminology in this persuasive argument. While in most cases of adoption it is clear that there are two distinct parties involved, the birth parents (e.g. the genetic father who had a sexual relationship with the genetic, birth mother) and the unrelated adoptive parents, with donor conception all these separate categories are entangled together. Most significantly there are no foundational birth parents and there is no relinquishing of a child they have produced together. With donor conception the birth mother is always the intended mother, even if she is not the genetic parent. If she conceives through sperm donation she is both genetic and birth mother and, most significantly, she has had no sexual connection with the donor, so there is no foundational sexual relationship with him. Her relationship is with her partner, who is also the intended father (or in the case of a lesbian couple, the second mother). If a woman conceives through egg donation then although she is not the genetic mother, she is both the biological and the birth mother (Konrad, 2005). That is to say she has nourished the embryo and caused it to grow and develop over nine months and she has also gone through the birth process and may breastfeed. When the sperm comes from her partner he is the genetic father and together they have a foundational relationship inasmuch as their union is the basis of the desire to have a child together. Donor conception parents are therefore not in the same shoes as adoptive parents and gamete donors do not have a relationship with the child born of their donation in the way that relinquishing parents have with their child (Jones and Hackett, 2012). The argument that donor conception should be treated in policy as if it were the same as adoption is therefore somewhat problematic (Haimes, 1988; Turkmendag, 2012).

Thinking about identity

There are a generation of children growing up today who do not know who they are.

(Turkmendag, 2012: 62)

These are the words of Julia Feast, speaking to BBC News in November 1998 in her capacity as project manager for the Children's Society, which was campaigning for a change in the law to donor conception to end donor anonymity. As Ilke Turkmendag has demonstrated, campaigning groups at the end of the 1990s and early 2000s focused a lot of attention on the idea of personal identity, which in turn was assumed to derive from correct knowledge about one's genetic forebears. This reasoning flows directly from the adoption debate and was captured particularly powerfully in the autobiographical account by Kate Adie (2005), whose book was titled *Nobody's Child: Who Are You When You Don't Know Your Past?* Adie was a foundling who was never able to trace her birth mother and she consequently argued that she had no roots in a tangible history which would have provided the ontological security that she was missing.

The idea of the theft of personal identity is a powerful trope which has a strong purchase in a contemporary popular imagination fuelled by programmes such as *Who Do You Think You Are?* (BBC) and *Long Lost Family* (ITV) or websites such as *Genes Reunited*. This approach tends to present identity as a fixed thing or cluster of attributes which are inherited through genetic connection but which cannot come to fruition without full knowledge of the person(s) from whom the genes derive. So, although it is the genetic connection that is seen to transport identity down the generations, it is implicit in the argument that full ontological security cannot be truly accessed unless the bearer of the genes is known in person. This understanding of identity rests heavily on the significance of personal histories and biography through which people can only understand who they 'really' are by knowing their correct lineage or roots (see Marshall, 2012). In other words identity is imagined as a kind of pearl hidden in an oyster which is known to be available but which can only be retrieved through the correct knowledge of one's ancestry. The idea that identity is linked to origins has a longstanding heritage. Although we suggest that this particular formulation of personal identity is problematic, it is also undeniably compelling. The idea of being embedded in a *proper* genealogical family tree, with an *accurate* family history and a *certainty* about who one's biological relatives are, is both comforting and alluring. By comparison, the opposite condition of being denied knowledge of one's origin can clearly give rise to a strong sense of dislocation and uncertainty (see also Carsten, 2004). This is one of the reasons why being illegitimate (or in English law 'the child of no one') used to be such a shameful condition. Not knowing one's father brought with it many problems and much adversity in the nineteenth and much of the twentieth century. Culturally speaking, being fatherless came to mean being 'nobody' and having few rights and a stigmatised status. Although all forms of legal discrimination against illegitimate persons have been abolished in the UK, there remains an undeniably significant cultural narrative (or script) about the importance of knowing one's origins. As Steph Lawler argues,

What is being expressed here is a deep sense of displacement. This seems to be related to a sense of *not knowing*, itself related to *not belonging*.

(2008: 42, emphasis in original)

However, the idea that personal identity resides exclusively in the knowledge of a specific genetic connection seems to stretch this narrative to an extreme. At the very least it tends to obliterate all the other factors that might contribute to the ongoing construction of personal identity. For example, migrants and refugees often point to the huge importance of place of origin for their identities, such that an identity as Barbadian or Mirpurian can become overwhelmingly important (Anderson, 2006; orig 1983). A specific language may also be seen as conferring identity according to campaigners for minority languages such as Welsh, such that the loss of a language in younger generations is seen as a loss of identity. A peer group may also provide a strong personal identity, especially for young people, as with subcultures such as goths or skinheads. At some points in a life course any of these sources of identity might become predominant and, in certain circumstances, one might develop into what Erving Goffman (1990) has referred to as a master status. In this situation a person may cleave to a single source of identity (e.g. ethnicity, religious adherence) to the exclusion of all others.

However, this does not mean that in the general course of events all people have only one defining personal identity. Most significantly for our argument here, we suggest that the family provides a particularly powerful personal identity relating to its unique mix of elements like social class, ethnicity, religion, cultural values, education, place and so on. It is only necessary to read a few autobiographical accounts of a life to recognise how important, even formative, people regard their early family experiences as being – whether for good or ill. Even such factors as birth order can be experienced as central to the formation of an individual identity and certainly being an only child or being the only girl among a tribe of boys can be experienced as very formative.

Once we start to understand identity in these more complex terms, the idea that there is one source to a 'real' and pre-eminent form of identity seems inadequate. Moreover, as Talja Bloklan (2005) has argued, identity is not a static thing which, once acquired, never changes. It is always in the process of becoming and in the process of being influenced by changing events and relationships. Her understanding of identity is that it is relational, which is to say that it is not that pearl in a shell that can be possessed and preserved unchanged; rather it ebbs and flows and changes (imperceptibly perhaps) in relation to the people one relates to in different contexts over time.

To understand identity as relational brings about an important conceptual shift. As Vanessa May (2013) argues, there is a tendency in Western cultures to see identity as an individual achievement and as flowing from internal, psychological processes. In this model identity is achieved by an individual as long as he or she is not denied the means to achieve their rightful identity. But a more sociological understanding of identity recognises that it can only be formed through relationships with others, at first mostly family members. In that context personal identity starts to be formed by the expectations of parents and relatives, then by the recognition of differences with others (e.g. having both a different gender and personality when compared with a brother or sister). These relationships then widen, such that experiences of sameness and difference occur in the playground, at university, at work and so on, forming complex webs of meaning and interpretation of the self. May goes on to argue that once we comprehend identity as relational, a better term to use for the field it tries to capture would be *belonging*. This is because the idea of belonging incorporates much more usefully the ways in which the individual is always located in a context made up of other people, material things and social structures, as well as more abstract notions such as nationality, ethnicity, gender, generation, heritage and so on. The feeling of belonging or not belonging is felt, often intensely, by an individual but that feeling is only possible because of the social connections and disconnections that give rise to the condition in the first place.

These insights into the meaning of belonging and identity add in important ways to our understanding of family life as a complex web of emotions, proximities, relationships, memories, biographies and various forms of connectedness. We see family practices (Morgan, 2011) such as daily forms of care, talking, play and housework as the fundamental stuff of making families, but we also recognise the crucial place of memory, connectedness and biography. This means that things like family stories (of a grandfather in a past war, of a mother's schooldays) are acknowledged as powerful in the process of creating the uniqueness of each family and also of creating memories to pass on to other generations. Family photographs or keepsakes, in this model of family life, are seen as material forms of connection (or sometimes disconnection) between kin and generations. In particular the family practice of spotting resemblances has emerged from this approach as a crucial way in which families bond together. Thus things like 'an uncle's nose' or 'a mother's mouth' are often rehearsed in families even though few family members may agree about such resemblances. But also less tangible qualities can be seen as a form of family resemblance (Mason, 2008). For example, a talent with a musical instrument might be attributed to a link with a cousin several times removed, or a taste for foreign travel may be seen as a connection with a great-grandparent who was a sailor. These acts of connection may rarely be literally 'true', indeed the way in which they are hotly contested in families suggests that they are unreliable at best. However, these discussions give rise to a sense of relatedness or belonging which appears to have a tangible basis, and which also have a powerful 'absent presence' in families of non-genetic connections (Becker *et al.*, 2005; Nordqvist, 2010).

We therefore suggest that family practices create relatedness. Of course in the majority of families this creation of relatedness and a sense of belonging maps onto genetic or biological kinship. Or at least we assume it does because, of course, we have no records of families in the past where children were not the genetic offspring of a father or where there were informal adoptions. But, putting that issue aside, the fact that these practices have appeared to map directly onto biological kinship has led to an understanding that biological or genetic links automatically give rise to a sense of bonding and belonging. Clearly the two phenomena are entangled, but we suggest that it is important to be able to distinguish between them. Following the work of anthropologists of kinship such as Janet Carsten (2004) and Jeanette Edwards (2000), and the work of sociologists Janet Finch and Jennifer Mason (1993), we suggest that there is now ample evidence to show that, on the one hand, genetic kinship does not automatically lead to caring, loving, close families and, on the other hand, family practices between non-genetic kin can give rise to bonding, security and a strong sense of belonging. These are not, of course, new ideas and we do not claim originality in restating them. But in the field of donor conception (and also adoption) there is a tendency for some of the more populist arguments to sweep aside all the evidence that exists on the importance of family practices in order to focus solely on genetic links, as if all the work that families do to create belonging, connectedness, biography and bonding is superfluous.

What we hope to demonstrate in the chapters that follow is the way in which the donor conceived families we interviewed for our study struggled to create precisely this sense of belonging for their children in the face of an increasingly unsympathetic popular culture that emphasises the predominance of genetic links. The starting point of all the couples we spoke to, whether lesbian or heterosexual, was their hope to have and raise children, and the older generation in the study also hoped to become grandparents. None of them was unaware of, or careless of, the fact that their children would not be solely genetically related to them. They struggled with the implications of this form of difference and were worried about what significance it might have for the lives of their children as they grew up. Many grandparents were worried about the idea of 'foreign' genes entering the family, and it is clear that most of our families had been influenced by populist thinking about the power of genes which left them uneasy in sometimes ill-defined ways. But the most important endeavour of both parents and grandparents was to ensure that the children 'belonged' in their families notwithstanding genetic difference. They wanted to give the children exactly the same things (in terms of love, attention, security) as other children in the family. As we note above, the grandparents and parents also wanted their families to be acknowledged as proper families, not as deviants whose choices and actions were dubious. For some this desired properness took the form of a close approximation to 'traditional' family forms, while for others the shape of properness was challenged to include a wider scope of kin and parenthood. In the chapters that follow we trace in detail how these families managed these issues and reveal the complex and sometimes very difficult decisions they have to take in their everyday family practices.

2
Uncharted Territories: Donor Conception in Personal Life

Introduction

In this chapter we explore the complex road that both heterosexual and lesbian couples traverse in the process of achieving a pregnancy against the odds. Of course the 'odds' facing heterosexual couples and lesbian couples are not exactly the same. Heterosexual couples only resort to assisted conception when they find out that one (or both) of them is infertile. This nearly always comes as a major upset. Lesbian couples do not experience this precise shock because, in wanting a child, they already know that they must take steps to secure sperm donation. However, they still have to undergo many medical procedures (if they go through clinics), they still have to make vital decisions about donation, and sometimes they also discover problems of infertility. There are also, of course, important gender differences which can significantly influence the distinct experiences of these couples. For these reasons we discuss the two groups separately, focusing initially on the heterosexual couples before turning to the lesbian couples. Although we will be emphasising the differences between them, where appropriate we shall also draw attention to overlapping issues and feelings.

Heterosexual couples and donor conception

When heterosexual couples enter into a serious relationship or marriage there is often a presumption that at some stage they will have children together. Indeed, at first, much effort may be put into preventing a pregnancy in order that a child or children will arrive at the right time and in the right circumstances. So the possibility (whether welcome or not) of creating a child together is often a fundamental element of such relationships. It is therefore little wonder that the inability to conceive is encountered as a profoundly adverse discovery.

In stating this we are, of course, not saying anything that is not already well known. However, there are specific components of this story that we want to focus on in order to understand the process that ends in donor conception. The first of these is the idea of 'having or making a child together'. The second is the loss of manhood associated with male infertility. The third is the desire to experience pregnancy and birth as a fundamental marker of womanhood. These elements become entangled in the process of decision-making and ultimately have a profound effect on how couples manage the transition from 'natural' conception to donor conception. They resonate through later reactions and responses to genetic and non-genetic links, to the 'inequality' between genetic and non-genetic parents, and to the idea of accommodating stranger genes into the family, which few of these parents ever imagined could happen.

Arriving at donor conception

> Holly: And then the doors keep closing, you have to look at different options.

With the exception of six couples who knew early on in their relationship that one of them was infertile or likely to be, the couples all embarked on the process of trying to conceive relatively optimistically. However, on discovering that they had problems, they began the process of fertility testing and ultimately assisted conception. This typically took the form of drug treatment (e.g. Clomid) to stimulate ovulation, IVF and/or ICSI. At this stage in the process the couples were totally committed to the idea that they would 'have a child together'. This commitment led many in our group of interviewees to have between 9 and 15 rounds of treatment and, because more than three rounds were not usually allowed on the NHS, many ended up spending thousands of pounds in the private sector (in one case £60,000 at 2011 values). The determination to have a child together meant that couples went through this treatment for a minimum of three years and sometimes for as many as ten years.

The huge emotional toll that undergoing infertility treatment takes on individuals and couples is now well documented (Franklin, 1997; Becker, 2000; Thompson, 2005) and the couples in our study were no exception to this. Although they all had children by the time we interviewed them, none had forgotten the ordeal they had gone through. The problem that they had faced was how to stop treatment and give up on the hope of having 'their own' child.

> Victoria: So there was this feeling of just wanting to move forward. And emotionally we [felt] we couldn't take much more IVF and…we said to the doctors, 'Well, you know, do you tell couples to stop ever?' And he said, 'Well, we sort of do advise.' And then I said something like, 'What would you say to us?' And he said, 'Well, yeah, you're probably coming to that point, yes, where we can't really say why it's not working, but it's not working.' We were at one of the best clinics in London, so we were throwing money at it and we'd had every test done and so then it was a case of, 'Right, what's next?' (212)

Victoria's experience was fairly typical because most couples simply became exhausted by the process, as well as finding themselves in financial difficulties. There were also problems of taking time off work for clinic appointments, not to mention the painful cycles of hope and despair. However, few of these couples moved easily from the ideal of creating a child together to the idea of donor conception. It was more typical for couples to think that their next step would be adoption and some began the process of finding out about adoption while others decided against it. The idea of donor conception as a 'middle way' came as something of a surprise to most. Initially many just rejected the idea out of hand. The feeling was that if the child was not going to be 'their' child, it would be better if there was no child at all, or that the child should be adopted so that it was the child of neither of them. This emphasis on complete togetherness was a crucial element in their thinking.

Thus, a further emotional transition was required to move couples beyond the idea of 'a child together' to the idea of a 'child of just one of us'. This process was often hastened by the 'biological clock' because after years of trying to conceive many of the women in our sample were in their late thirties or in some cases just over 40, and so they felt they had little time left. But in spite of the ominous ticking, couples could take at least a year and sometimes longer to come to terms with the idea of donor conception. It was not something decided upon easily and it entailed dispensing with cherished hopes and ideals. This was due to a complex interweaving of concerns and emotions, many of which were linked to notions of manhood and womanhood.

Manhood

> Trevor: I turned to her [the counsellor] and I said 'Well how do you deal with this stuff?' She said 'The truth is you don't, you kind of, you live with it.' Which was a nice sort of thing, and I think [it] helped me massively, that speech. It means you don't have to come out the other side and everything be okay, you just live with it and you deal with it and you try and let it affect you as little as possible and more appropriately at the right times when it, kind of when it should affect you, rather than just kind of putting on stuff which actually has got nothing to do with it. (213)

> Carrie: I mean I don't [know] how much you want me to say [about how my husband reacted] but you know he's said to me... at the time of the counselling and since then, he sort of buries a lot of it. But I think he's still got unresolved issues about it. (208)

> Joshua: You know [male infertility] is becoming more and more of an issue. And I think it's not something men talk about. Because it's, you know, I suppose the grieving part of it is... it does feel in a way as if, in some way, you're less of a man because you can't produce kids, and it's kind of a bit silly in a way really, but it's the emotional kind of feeling, I think. (206)

In our sample of 22 heterosexual couples, 13 received sperm donation and 9 received egg donation. Of those needing to receive sperm, four of the men knew from childhood or adolescence that they were infertile because they had experienced cancer or other serious illnesses. These men felt that they had come to terms with the issue of infertility gradually over many years and so they were prepared for donor conception when the time came. A further man had had a vasectomy which could not be reversed and a final man had had mumps later in life but had fathered one child 'naturally', but then the couple had to turn to donor conception for subsequent children. This left seven men who had to face the complete shock of infertility later in life. They all found it incredibly difficult to handle, as the passages of quotation above indicate. Two of the men who found it particularly difficult opted not to be interviewed by us and so the reports we have about their reactions come from their partners, but the remaining five did speak personally about their feelings, their anger and their grief.

It was not always clear what these men were most angry or distressed about. Clearly the most significant problem for them was their inability to father a child and this could mean that they felt less of a man. But they also felt great distress at not being able to give their wives the thing that they most craved, namely a pregnancy and a child. This was therefore a double disappointment because not only did they feel that they 'let themselves down' as men, but they also let their partners down. Mixed in with these feelings too was an anger about the silence surrounding male infertility. Trevor, for example, seemed enraged by the fact that infertility treatment was all about women and he was angry that (as he saw it) there were no support groups for men. He felt invisible and alone with his distress. However, other couples seemed to find a partial solution to the problem of men's distress that husbands were largely ignored in the process and that their wives were typically assumed to be the ones with the fertility trouble. And some men said that the last thing they wanted to do was talk to other men about it. They felt that their friends would not understand and would just be embarrassed if such a topic was raised. So, many of these men suffered alone, even finding it hard to tell their own fathers about their infertility.

The men often found themselves in a kind of Catch-22 situation. If they expressed their anger and rage at their infertility then they felt (regardless of whether it was true or not) that there was a risk that their partners would be denied donor sperm because they had 'unresolved issues'. This is because all couples have to go through a process of counselling prior to donor conception and there was a worry that they could be turned down if they were deemed unsuitable. But if they presented themselves as entirely accepting of the situation and the proposed solution, they felt they could not speak openly about what they were going through. In a way they were forced to restrain their feelings for the sake of their wives, most of whom had been trying for years to get pregnant. James expresses this predicament most clearly:

> James: So I thought, 'Well, let's go and find out about it then,' because I'm sitting here totally against [sperm donation] but that's purely...Neanderthal man talking. 'Let's try and look at this a bit more sensibly and go against what my instinct is telling me.' So I just started going to the [support group] and met some really nice people and found it amazing that there were guys that were just completely open to it and accepting and were right up for it and couldn't wait to get started. And I was going, 'Are you for real?'...And for me, it was a case of, 'Well, I've either got to go with this or not. Let's look a little bit further into the – into the future. What does it hold if we do this route or that route?' And as painful as it was – I mean, emotionally, I was distraught. I hated it. It was soul destroying....I think I just draw a blank on that now, other than it raises its ugly head now and again....You know, it's that – it's – it's the grief, I think. I grieved a lot for the child I'll never have, blah, blah, blah. It's like talking to my counsellor now. (203)

James stopped going to the support group because he found himself so out of step with the other men there. What was interesting, however, was that he really did not believe that the other hopeful fathers were content with the predicament they were in. He felt strongly that they were putting on a mask to make things all right for their partners and to make themselves acceptable in the therapeutic environment. We have, of course, no way of knowing if James was correct in his reading of the situation. It might have been, for example, that some of the men in his group had had childhood illnesses, which meant that they had indeed come to terms with their infertility. But James might also have intuited something profound because of all the seven men we know of who found out about their infertility late in life (and when in a permanent relationship) none were easy with their situation and some openly expressed worries for the future.

Womanhood

> Erin: So yeah, so there's the sort of grieving and the kind of... the sort of loss of this kind of future that you've got in your mind's eye and I think also, for me there was a huge sense of failure I just felt, I can't do this, you know, this is something that everybody else appears to be able to do, which of course isn't true but it feels like it at the time, and I felt a massive failure. I just, I really, really struggled with that and I felt angry and cross with the world and cross with myself and just so sort of, you know, I didn't know where to go with any of it. So I did really struggle. (217)

It was evident that the women felt just as acute a sense of failure as did the men. Our interviews with grandparents (which are discussed in the next chapter) lend support to this too because it was often the case that daughters had to rely on their mothers (and sometimes mothers-in-law) at such times and the full weight of their grieving was felt by the older generation (Nordqvist and Smart, forthcoming 2014). While our sense was that the men did not share their own anguish except in a limited way with their partners, the women shared theirs with parents (particularly mothers) and close friends. The women were therefore more supported, but they were of course the ones going for all the tests, taking the drugs, having the treatments and so on. While some men who were infertile had to undergo some tests (and in one case an operation), it tended to be their wives who were spending endless days going back and forth to clinics, often accompanied by their mothers because the men were at work.

What also became clear was that it was the women who were most driven in their desire to become parents. So while the men suffered from the knowledge of their own infertility or were hugely disappointed if their wives were infertile, we gained the strong impression that it was the women who were driving the process forward and who were unwilling to give up 'too easily'. Often it seemed that the men put themselves in the position of the supportive prop and would be willing to go along with whatever their wives wanted because they acknowledged that ultimately the consequences seemed so much more devastating for the women.

In our sample of 22 heterosexual couples, nine received egg donation. As we suggest above, they did not rush to donation as a simple or easy solution to their childlessness. The women agonised over whether it was ethically correct to receive donor gametes or whether it would bring long-term problems for the children conceived in this way. In an approach that mirrored men's worries about raising 'another man's child', so too the women worried about giving birth to 'another woman's baby'. However, an important difference between the genders arose at this point in the couple's reasoning because it became clear that although the women we spoke to grieved over their inability to have 'their own' children as a couple, they found comfort in the idea that they could still become pregnant and give birth. Gamete donation gave them the promise of all the real experiences of motherhood and although they grieved for the loss of genetic links, they were consoled by the experience of gestation, birth and lactation (Konrad, 2005).

> Melissa: So I felt that lack of being a woman you know, that was a very strong feeling initially, but being pregnant I felt like I was helping make that baby, so a third part of the cog. (216)
> Adrian: And also – I know Elizabeth also really wanted to carry her own child and that was very important for her. (221)
> Zoe: It was at that point that we were talking about different ways of having a family, wasn't it, about adoption? We looked into that and then decided that we would like to, you know, go through a pregnancy. And, you know, to have our own children that way. So we went the donor route, didn't we? (202)

For some of the women in the heterosexual sample the achievement of a pregnancy was described as something that healed their suffering and gave them a proper future as a mother. But for others a pregnancy was about the couple. Thus Zoe in the final quotation above says that they decided that *they* would like to go through a pregnancy. The period of gestation was clearly seen by many women as a healing period, especially where there had been sperm donation. And many referred to the fact that the couple together would have a newborn baby to raise together 'from day one'.

Clinging to togetherness was therefore really important for these couples, and this idea was mobilised to overcome the deep-seated worry that the child they would produce would be genetically related to only one of them.

Holly: It won't be my genetic child. [I found that] terribly hard, terribly hard, it wouldn't be our child and because we conceived two babies naturally and they were never going to be born clearly – [due to miscarriage]... it felt, because [the egg donor] is a very good friend, it did feel, for a while, that it was like my husband and my best friend were sleeping together even though it wasn't like that. But, it felt like they were going to have an intimate relationship to produce a baby that I would carry. (218)

The existence of a third party, the donor, troubled the automatic presumption that these couples had held that having a baby was just about the two of them. It also introduced an element of inequality between them because while one parent had the (perceived) security of genetic connection, the other did not. We explore the significance of this idea of genetic connection in Chapters 7 and 8, but here it is important to acknowledge that at the stage of embarking on donor conception, the heterosexual couples were all very worried about what this genetic imbalance (as they saw it) would bring.

Coming to terms with it

Brenda: I didn't feel the baby would be mine. I felt I would be taking a baby from somebody else. I felt very strongly about that.... It was a very odd feeling, you know, to be using someone's eggs. And I saw these eggs as children, I didn't see them as just eggs, as bits of tissue, I actually saw them as real children. (211)

Cara: I was carrying a sort of a slightly alien being, which you feel anyway when you're pregnant because you don't know who or what it's going to be, if you like. But there was this extra element of anonymity about it. (220)

These two quotations capture some of the anxieties that the women who were pregnant from gamete donation felt. Cara, who had conceived her first child 'naturally', had the experience to recognise that any pregnancy can feel a bit alien, but nonetheless both Brenda and Cara refer to a kind of strangeness about not knowing the full origins of the child they were carrying. The child, many feared, would be a kind of stranger rather than a (supposedly) predictable melange of known genes or characteristics and features. However, over time, these feelings did dissipate to a certain extent. It would not be accurate to suggest that they vanished entirely with the birth of a child or children, because so many parents referred to a kind of lingering, but relatively mild, qualm. However, all of the parents stated forcefully that once they had their children they were glad that they had pursued donor conception. As Daniel and Robert put it below, once a relationship develops with the child, previous anxieties seem to fade:

> Daniel: (To be honest) it's not something that really, you know, it's not something I feel on a day to day basis at all because there's such a real relationship. (201)
> Robert: I don't find myself wishing they were genetically my children. I mean, I agree that would have been [nice].
> Jennifer: If, if I could take these two and, yes, change their history so that you were their genetic father then that would be fine,
> Robert: Yes, yes, but...
> Jennifer: But I wouldn't wish to, you know. I wouldn't wish to have different children than I have now. So, you have to say what we did was what was right for us and, you know, it's worked out for the best. (210)

Real-life, everyday activities of loving and caring for a child came to weigh more heavily in the balance for these parents than their previous, more abstract concerns about whose genes were inherited. However, we are not suggesting that these issues disappear altogether, and we explore them more fully later.

Lesbian couples and donor conception

The process of having a child by donor conception is experienced by heterosexual parents as something like getting to the finishing line of a particularly difficult obstacle race. For lesbian parents it was also an obstacle course, but the hurdles were not the same and called for different emotional and personal resources to reach the finishing line. As we note above, the lesbian couples were prepared for difficulties once they decided they wanted to become parents. They knew their choices were either adoption (although this was a relatively recent choice for couples when we conducted our interviews) or sperm donation. There was therefore no anguish about the unfairness of being unable to conceive 'naturally' and the motif of grief, which was so strong among the heterosexual couples, was virtually absent with the lesbian couples. This meant that these interviews were far less harrowing and much more focused on practicalities and ethical decision-making. So the obstacle course facing the lesbian couples consisted of questions of how to go about finding sperm donors, whether to use informal processes or clinics (and if so how to find a clinic that would offer treatment to a lesbian couple) and whether to involve a known donor or opt for a completely anonymous donation.

In theory (because, as we shall show, actual practice is different) couples could choose between a number of options. One option was to receive sperm donation at a clinic where the donor would be unknown to them but whose identity could be revealed to a child when he or she reached 18 years of age. Secondly, they could find a sperm donor from among their friends or acquaintances, creating not only a known donor but possibly an involved father figure for their child. Thirdly, they could take their known donor through the clinic system, which would mean that he would abandon legal claims to paternity and the child might not discover his identity until reaching the age of 18. Fourthly, they could find an anonymous donor through the Internet, never know anything about him and have virtually no contact with him. Finally, like heterosexual couples, they could go abroad to a clinic where there would be safeguards in terms of the quality of sperm they received (or possibly for egg donation) and where complete anonymity could still be achieved. The kinds of choices facing these couples can be envisaged with the help of the matrix below (Figure 2.1).

The basic choices they faced were therefore between known/ identity release donor or a completely anonymous donor (shown on the left-right axis in the diagram) and between home or clinic conception (shown on the up-down axis in the diagram). In practice what we found, however, was that these were not always *real* choices because, for example, some couples could not afford to pay the fees of private clinics while others could not find a willing donor who wanted to become a father figure to a subsequent child. This meant that the choice between home and clinic conception was highly constrained. Moreover, some couples started by wanting to go down one route only to find that they had to change direction or that they changed their views as they gained more knowledge. Thus a preferred

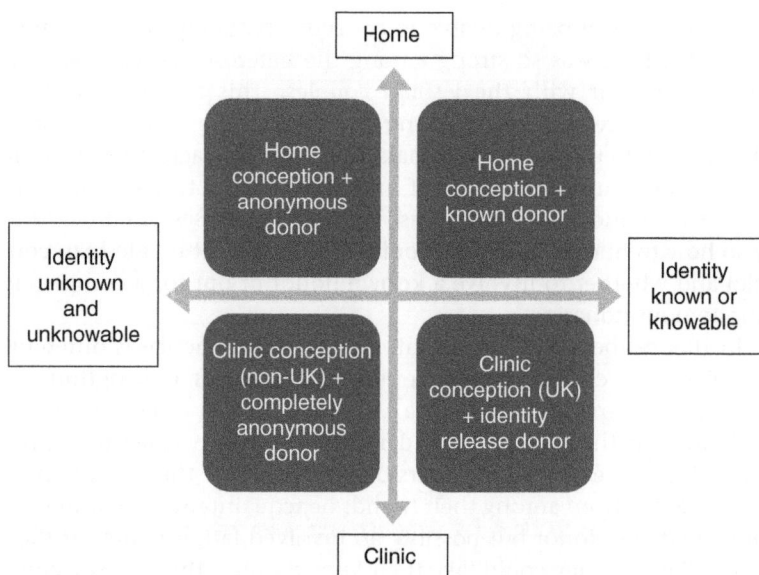

Figure 2.1 Visualising dimensions of 'choice'

home conception with a known donor might encounter unexpected problems, meaning that the couple would end up in a clinic because it could offer much greater legal protection. In yet other situations, some couples might have one child by one route, but a second child via another because circumstances (e.g. local policy or national legislation) had changed. In asking couples about their plans for having children we therefore found that they could tell clear stories about their original strategies, but as the stories unfolded we learnt how these simple plans had to be jettisoned as they progressed across the obstacle course. In what follows we explore some of the key elements in the process, focusing mainly on decisions about known or anonymous donors. Finally we explore decisions about which partner would actually get pregnant because we found that this was also a significant decision for the couples.

Anonymous donors preferred

Sharon: I accept that all family units are different now, but I don't know, it just, for us it seemed best that it was anonymous and that there wasn't a third wheel kind of, cause I don't know, even if, with the best will in the world and if they're your closest friend, you're still not going to see eye to eye on things and, I don't know, I think that would be messy and you know not the best thing for a child I suppose, in my particular opinion. (118)

Sharon stressed the thing that was so important to many lesbian mothers, namely that they should feel safe in their position as the parents of their children. They wanted to be able to make decisions without a third party having a say or interfering. She also clearly felt that there should be only two parents and argued that cases she knew of where there were three or even four involved parents/parent-figures 'blew her mind' and could not be in the best interests of the children. Unfortunately some couples 'opted' for anonymity because they felt they had no other choice:

Jenny: So we went with an anonymous donor because we liter-ally ran out of options. It's not as if we had all these choices, 'Oh which one shall we have?' It wasn't like that. (121)

Some couples simply could not afford the cost of donor insemination in private clinics and so were, in a sense, forced onto the unregulated market (e.g. through the Internet). Others simply could not find a friend or relative who would be willing to donate even though they wanted their child to know their donor. Yet others found they had to go abroad because they needed egg donation as well as sperm dona-tion and in so doing had to accept that their children would not be able to trace their donors.

Known donors preferred

Known donors fall into three categories. The first type is the identity release donor who provides sperm through a UK clinic. The second type is the donor who provides sperm through a clinic but who is already known to the recipients. This means that the couple will know a lot about the donor and may even involve him in the life of the child. However, as we point out above, the couple benefit from all the legal protections governing their parenthood that the clinical process currently provides. That is to say they alone will be recog-nised as the legal parents of the child. Finally, there is the known donor who donates sperm informally and who is therefore, in English law, the father of the child. In these cases, although the legal status of the birth mother is secure, the birth mother's partner may not be automatically recognised as a parent if they are not in a civil partnership/marriage. It is these cases that have led to a number of legal disputes over the rights of the genetic father to have contact with the child and to share in decision-making concerning the child's upbringing (we discussed one such case in Chapter 1). What this all means, therefore, is that when lesbian couples opt for a known donor they still have to consider what degree of closeness should be entailed.

The core principle in favour of known donors (of any degree) is the idea that a child should be able to know 'where s/he comes from'.

> Angela: You know, we consulted friends and family and, you know, ... they had different opinions and some of them said, 'Oh, yeah, you know, that's absolutely fine. You want your family.' And then some said, 'Well, if you can choose to know the father, why would you then choose not to know the father?' (107)
> Jenny: I had this image of this child asking me 'Who is my dad?' and me saying 'We don't know and you will never know,' and I really didn't want to do that. (121)

The idea of opting for a known donor was therefore a matter of principle and basically reflected an adherence to the idea of the rights of the child to know about their origins (Donovan, 2000; Nordqvist, 2012b). In some instances couples wanted the donor to be involved with the child at least to the extent that he would be a fairly familiar figure in the child's life. In the case of Laura and Natalie, where the donor would be more distant, they had created a memory book for their son with all sorts of details about the donor. The memory book is akin to the method used in adoption processes and is seen as a way to make absent parent(s) more tangible as well as preserving a memory which might otherwise be lost.

The desire to find a willing donor who met criteria such as height, colouring or age as well as being willing to be a 'family friend' or 'sort of uncle' was often unachievable, however. Some couples were frankly just lucky. So Bridget and Lori did not even have to ask because a heterosexual married couple they were friendly with offered them the husband's sperm. But Miranda and Jenny spent over a decade looking for such a donor and in the end had to give up and go to a clinic. Fortunately for them, by the time they entered into the clinical process the law had changed and their donor had opted into the identity release scheme so at least they had the comfort of knowing that their daughter (who was born the year the law changed in 2005) would be able to access information about her donor. Other couples were not so lucky and, although they may have wanted known donors, found themselves (prior to 2005) in a situation where their children's donors were quite anonymous.

It is important to acknowledge the significance of the passage of time in order to understand how it was that these couples could change their minds about having a known donor. As with the heterosexual couples, the biological clock was ticking for the lesbian mothers. For many it was a matter of sticking with their original ideals and giving up the idea of having children, or adjusting their point of view because the main priority was to achieve a pregnancy and to produce a child. Thus many of the couples reflected ruefully on their early aspirations. For example, they may have had very clear ideas about the type of donor they wanted whether in terms of physical appearance, personality or education and employment profiles. But when faced with either very little choice of donors or having waited years for the right one, they willingly settled for something different. This could also mean that some couples went abroad for a donor, especially for egg donation. This decision arose typically because of the problem of the biological clock and the fact that waiting for egg donation in the UK could take years (after having spent many years in the system already). But this often combined with the fact that the treatment was considerably cheaper abroad and, when couples were faced with the possibility of needing several cycles of treatment, such economic decisions were not based on simple preferences. This meant that some parents went for anonymous donors even though it was not what they wanted for their children, justifying the decision on the basis that otherwise there would be no children at all.

Choosing the birth mother

In one very significant regard the lesbian mothers we interviewed had an advantage over the heterosexual couples because, in theory at least, they could choose which parent would be the birth mother. This meant that there was an ideal possibility of both parents becoming birth parents should they decide to have more than one child because both mothers could conceive, carry the pregnancy and give birth to children genetically related to them. This provided the possibility of a kind of perfect equality which was very attractive to the parents. However, the reality did not always match the ideal because sometimes a significant age difference might mean that one partner was 'too old' to conceive or, at least, felt that they had gone beyond the stage of wanting to be pregnant and give birth themselves.

> Linda: ... and I always knew that I wanted to have children. I think Dawn had got to the stage in her life where she had ...
> Dawn: No intention.
> Linda: ... accepted she wasn't going to have any and no intention of having them. (111)

With some couples one partner wanted children more than the other and so it was agreed that only one would conceive, while in others infertility was discovered, which meant that only one could get pregnant before both biological clocks reached midnight. Sometimes the consequences of assisted reproduction meant plans had to change:

> Jessica: So I was going to get pregnant and potentially Amy was [going to] later but I had IVF treatment after a couple of goes at IUI [intrauterine insemination] which was ...
> Amy: Yeah four cycles of IUI first.
> Jessica: So and then because I gave birth to twins we've then not had any more and I don't think we would have. We didn't save any of the sperm we were given which was probably a mistake but I think we'd already decided that we probably were having two and that would be it. (101)

Our interviews with the lesbian couples revealed them to be far more relaxed about issues of genetic parentage than the heterosexual couples, who often seemed consumed with grief and anxiety about the issue. The lesbian mothers seemed merely to be practical and while the ideal might have been for both to give birth to children, if this did not materialise it did not seem to generate an emotional crisis or burden of grief. There may have been disappointment but this seemed to be heavily outweighed by the arrival of children in their families. Sometimes extra steps were taken just to ensure that the non-birth mother did not feel excluded. So, for example, when Julia gave birth it was really important for her that the children took her partner's surname as a way of balancing out the fact that they had her genes. However, what often materialised as a more significant worry for the non-birth mother was the possibility that a known sperm donor would be treated as the father of their children and as more important than them. So the anxieties that arose seemed less about bonding with a child and more about the possibility that a donor could usurp their position in the family. Such worries were not without foundation, especially if the couple were not in a civil partnership or if the child was born before the non-birth mother was able to have her name legally included on the birth certificate as a 'female parent', a possibility in the UK since 2009. A significant number of lesbian parents who conceived prior to this date and who had gone through informal sperm donation had to adopt their children to safeguard their legal position. This entailed acquiring the formal permission of the sperm donor, who had to agree to be interviewed by social workers before he could give up his legal parentage. It was therefore little wonder that non-birth mothers might feel insecure, and in at least one case the couple had not proceeded with adoption because they were worried about the effect it might have on the donor if he was asked to relinquish his legal standing. In other instances, depending on the date of birth of subsequent children, a non-birth mother could find she had to go through the process of adopting an older sibling while she was automatically recognised as the parent of subsequent children born after changes to the law.

> Julia: We were very clear cut that we wanted Molly to be a full parent in law and in everything else ... and she had to go through the adoption process with Jack, which took about eight months, so she's now a full legal parent to Jack. Fortunately with Eve, the law has caught up so she can go straight on the birth certificate for Eve. But for Jack, we actually had to go through the adoption, so we had to have a social worker and references and lots and lots of meetings with the social worker and we had to go to court for her to be granted, you know, legal rights as a parent. (103)

Conclusion

It is clear from the accounts of both heterosexual and lesbian parents who have resorted to donor conception that the cultural and personal meanings of so doing are widely different. In the case of heterosexual parents the resort to gamete donation is enveloped in a pall of failure and dismay, at least for those who expect to be able to conceive naturally. Donor conception signifies not only infertility but also ultimately the extinguishing of one genetic line of inheritance and this is seen as a basis for much grief and regret. The counselling process that heterosexual couples go through frames their experiences of donor conception in terms of a bereavement, and feelings of grief are affirmed as akin to the loss of a child. We found many of the heterosexual couples we interviewed used exactly this kind of terminology to express their feelings and many also anticipated that they would never fully come to terms with their loss, in much the same way that it is now understood that one never comes to terms with the death of a loved one. The heterosexual experience is therefore framed almost exclusively in terms of loss.

In stark contrast, the lesbian experience is framed in terms of an (often unexpected) opportunity. For these parents gamete donation is wonderfully fortuitous and it is experienced in terms of a positive measure that allows them to create the family they want. The majority of the lesbian parents also wanted their children to know about their donor and to be able to contact them later on, if they were not in touch throughout their childhoods. Of course, it is true that the lesbians were not in a position to obscure the origins of the children they had given birth to, but they seemed to positively embrace the idea of known donors – with the proviso that their family unit was protected against undue interference. While the heterosexual couples were also mostly prepared to tell their children about their origins (see Chapters 4 and 5) none seemed to think it was a good idea that their children should know their sperm[1] donors throughout their childhood. To put it simply, for heterosexual parents the decision to resort to donor conception was conceptualised as a glass half empty, while for lesbian parents it was seen as a glass half full. Both had to achieve pregnancy and parenthood against the odds and lesbian parents often had the additional burden of encountering varying degrees of homophobia in the process, but the framing of the experience was completely different for the different sets of couples. The possible exception to this pattern was those heterosexual parents who had come to terms with infertility in childhood; they were much more likely to adopt a practical and pragmatic view of the process.

Donor conception was therefore, in practice, not a simple step for any of our parents. Even if it was not accompanied by feelings of grief and loss, hard choices had to be made. But thus far we have discussed the parents as if they existed in a tiny bubble of just two people without any outside influences, networks of support or family pressures. In actuality this could not be further from the truth and so in the next chapter we turn to look at the context of the wider family in which these couples were operating to gain a better understanding of the complex dynamics at work where genetically unrelated children are brought into families.

3
Ripples through the Family

Introduction

In this chapter our focus is on how the decision to conceive a child from donor gametes can have the kind of effect that a pebble has when dropped into a small pond. That is to say the decision causes ripples that spread out from the couple to impact upon wider family relationships. These ripples may be gentle nudges but at times they may seem like tiny tsunamis which threaten the equilibrium of the extended family. It is our argument that assisted reproduction in general, and donor conception specifically, occurs within a complex network of relationships and is not simply a matter for the central couple. Although the science of assisted conception necessarily concentrates on the couple (and often this narrows to a focus on the woman who carries the pregnancy) the experience of seeking a pregnancy 'against the odds' takes place within pre-existing family relationships and often with family members attending at a slight distance or offering substantial support and commentary. The nature of the support offered to couples going through the process can vary greatly, but the point is that we should not ignore its significance. When a donor conceived child is born he or she is not just born to the couple but born into a wider family and into a set of multifaceted connections. He or she is also born into a group of kin or a family lineage, will take a family name and will also carry forward the hopes of the next generation. The birth of the child therefore involves a wide range of folk with those closest to the first ripple most affected and those further away, like cousins or distant aunts and uncles, perhaps hardly touched at all or only fleetingly. While it may seem rather trite to emphasise this fact we suggest that these other important 'players' are often forgotten in research and writing on assisted reproduction. So much focus is placed on the couple with the fertility problems, or the woman who is desperate to conceive, that it appears as if only they matter. Their support networks are often ignored or simply taken for granted and yet, as we will show in subsequent chapters, family networks are hugely significant in playing a part in how knowledge of (and information about) donor conception is managed in families.

We explore these ripples through the family in two ways. First we examine what happens during the phase when couples are making decisions about donor conception and are undergoing treatment. In this discussion we will focus on the importance of family support. Then we explore what happens to these relationships once the child is born. As we will show, it is often at that point that the views and attitudes of the different generations are most divergent. As mentioned in Chapter 2, we found that the experiences of the heterosexual couples and the lesbian couples were often quite dissimilar. They faced different levels of support and, most significantly, how families responded to the birth of a child could be quite different. This means that once again we discuss these parents separately in order to give sufficient attention to their different experiences. Following the pattern of the previous chapter, we start with the heterosexual parents.

Phase one: Getting pregnant

a) The families of heterosexual couples

As we discuss in Chapter 2, one of the main issues for the heterosexual couples was coming to terms with infertility because, with the exception of a few of the men who knew that childhood illnesses had caused infertility, for most couples it came as a complete shock. It follows therefore that it was also something of a blow to the parents of these couples who were hoping to become grandparents. Clearly some of them had invested a great deal in anticipating the arrival of grandchildren and were either dropping hints or simply waiting to hear the good news. One of the grandmothers we interviewed explained that she was accompanying her daughter while she was house hunting and she kept advising against houses which she thought were unsuitable for a growing family.

> Wendy: So I kept saying 'Well this house wouldn't be any use,...,because there's nowhere to put a pram.' And eventually she said to me 'Mum, will you please not keep saying this because we're not having any children, we can't have any children.' (405)

From the moment of knowing that a daughter (or her partner) was infertile the parents, or more typically the mothers, were cast in the role of supporter-in-chief. Support usually flowed from mother to daughter, even where it was the male partner who was infertile, simply because it was the daughter who needed to get pregnant and had to attend the clinics, take the drugs and face the monthly anticipation of failure. (We say something about support for sons below). The mother–daughter bond, especially where it had been strong anyway, became almost vice-like for some. Some daughters phoned their mothers on a daily basis when treatment was intense; mothers could even be the first to know if there was another failure. In other cases mothers attended clinic appointments with their daughters (and sometimes daughters-in-law) because husbands or partners were at work. The problem of infertility could come to completely dominate the lives of the older as well as the younger generation. These comments from grandparents sum up their experiences:

> Lisa: I think for those, for those three or four years or whatever it was, about three years I suppose, while – while they were making the decision. . . . I had to – personally it was my biggest issue in life. (410)
> Sally: Well, I've been with [daughter] from the beginning over it, so over all her failed [attempts], everything. (411)
> Frances: So as far as I was concerned, yes, I didn't go through it all with her each time but if it didn't happen, then she would be upset and give me a call. (413)
> Petra (interviewer): And...at which point did she talk to you about this?
> Shirley: All the way through. (409)

The primacy of the mother–daughter bond does not mean that fathers were indifferent or unsupportive towards daughters. Often their role was mediated by their wives and sometimes their prime concern was to support their wives in supporting their daughters.

Their support was also often vital when it came to offering financial assistance. Given the high cost of repeated cycles of infertility treatment over many years it was often essential that parents contributed towards the costs.

> Barbara: I mean, we've actually funded two rounds of IVF.
> William: Yeah.
> Barbara: So we have been very (laughter) involved with all that. (406)
> Roger: If money is an issue we will bend over backwards to find money. (410)

While the parents of daughters seemed to become intensely involved in the struggle to conceive, the parents of infertile sons seemed to play a smaller role. This is not to suggest that these parents were uncaring but it seems to reflect the nature of parent–son relationships and the shape they assumed before the problem of infertility was manifest. Infertile sons seemed not to want to call on their parents for support and in turn the parents seemed not to know how to offer it. This might have been the outcome of what were regarded as proper relationships with independent adult sons and in one case the middle-class trope of the 'stiff upper lip' was mobilised to explain the lack of responsiveness.

> Carrie: The piece of the jigsaw we're not sure about in a way is Paul's parents, because they're not genetically related to [our child] you know. And I don't really know what they think about it. They're quite sort of a little bit stiff upper lip really, very British (laughter). (208)

The parents-in-law of infertile men also found it hard to know what to say or do to offer support, often because it was feared that any attempt would be experienced as demeaning. Put simply, the ordeal of infertility created a carpet of egg shells on which families had to tread.

The fact that the lives of the older generation could become so consumed with the problems of infertility could have consequences for other relatives and kin as well. Looking after a daughter, perhaps over several years, could mean that other children or relatives were neglected. For example, Roger and Lisa encountered problems with Roger's sister because during the period when their daughter was trying to conceive, Roger's mother developed increasingly severe dementia. Roger's sister began to feel increasingly burdened with her care and with the responsibility of arranging her affairs and felt that Roger was letting her down. She basically criticised him and Lisa for 'sitting comfortably down in the West Country' while she was being run ragged by their mother's condition. What Roger's sister did not know, because Roger and Lisa had had to keep it a secret, was that they were going up and down to London with their daughter to attend clinical appointments and they had no space at all in which to fit additional caring responsibilities. Once the situation was explained, Roger's sister could understand, but the impact on the wider family was substantial. There were many other examples of family relationships becoming strained. It was, for instance, particularly problematic when a sister (or sister-in-law) became pregnant at the same time as the infertile couple were still trying to conceive.

> Sally: So all that time it was only me who knew. So I had to keep sort of, you know, shelving my mother off and my sister, and it took a toll I have to say, because [my daughter] was terrible. . . . And every time anybody got pregnant . . . when her sister got pregnant she was sick. [My daughter] was physically sick when she knew that [her sister] was pregnant. It was just awful. I mean it just tore my family apart actually. (411)
>
> Lisa: And after they came back [from abroad] I think [my daughter] expected to conceive immediately because her identical twin sister had conceived one month after she'd got married. (410)

Speaking from the point of view of a sister, Nina, who was one of the lesbian mothers we interviewed, told us how difficult her relationship with her heterosexual sister became because the latter could not get pregnant.

> Nina: I've got an older sister. She's six years older than me. And it was difficult 'cause she's had difficulty conceiving. So she's been trying to get pregnant for about three years now. . . . So it kind of made the whole thing very tense with my sister because she's

just in such a difficult position really and she thought she would be the first person, you know, she thought she'd get pregnant immediately and it wouldn't be a problem for her and she'd be the one that has the first grandchild and all of those things. And obviously [she thought] that I wouldn't have children because I'm in a same-sex relationship. (116)

In another example one of the men we interviewed found it particularly difficult that his younger brother had fathered children before he had succeeded (as he saw it) in getting his wife pregnant. For these siblings the problem was not simply that they could not have children when their brothers or sisters could, but that the 'natural' order of things was painfully upset when a younger sibling overtook them in the race to turn their parents into grandparents.

Sometimes couples undergoing infertility treatment would refuse to attend family gatherings because they could not handle being with other relatives who had children. In turn this could mean that grandparents ceased to host such events or it could mean that relationships became strained because the couple in question would not tell anyone else why they were failing to turn up to family events. It was particularly hard for some mothers who felt they could not rejoice in the pregnancy of one daughter because their other daughter was unable to conceive. Thus infertility could cast a pall over the whole wider family and what could make it particularly difficult was that only a handful of relatives knew the cause of the chill that had descended.

b) The families of lesbian couples

As we discussed in Chapter 2, donor conception tended to be regarded as a positive opportunity for lesbian couples and not a poor or difficult alternative to 'natural conception'. This meant that when the couples embarked on the process of donor conception they were not usually in need of emotional support from their parents. If they did begin to encounter infertility problems, however, then this situation could change and mothers could find that they were brought in to support their daughters in exactly the same way as the mothers of heterosexual children.

In many ways the process of going for donor conception in lesbian based families was the complete antithesis of what it meant for heterosexual-based families. In the latter the decision was shrouded in the despair of infertility and often came after years of trying IVF and drug treatments. But for the former it was simply a positive step on the road to having children. Indeed for the parents of lesbians it was often thrilling news, as so many had assumed that they could never have grandchildren because their daughters were in a same-sex relationship. Many of the lesbians we interviewed spoke of the grief of their parents (particularly mothers) on being told that they were gay, but they pointed to the fact that this grief was often largely about the perceived loss of grandchildren.

> Nina: I can remember when I came out to my mum. It was one of the things that she really cried about, was, I won't have grandchildren, you know, I won't have children and she won't have grandchildren from me. And I think that was probably more of a loss for her than many other things associated with, you know, with my coming out and being gay. So, when we started talking about getting pregnant and having a baby [she was delighted]. (116)

The parents of lesbian couples we interviewed also confirmed this general view, namely that coming out was interpreted as a kind of familial or even genetic 'dead-end' which they mourned. Therefore, on discovering that it was no such thing, they were very enthusiastic about the procedure of donor conception.

> Judith: And I looked at her and said, then she repeated it and then I...I kind of, I just screamed, I said 'Oh oh' you know, I said, 'That's fantastic', I had tears in my eyes, I'm getting all teary again now. It was just really exciting, yes. (305)

It was the case, however, that the older generation often knew little about the procedures involved. Lesbian couples tended not to involve their parents in the ongoing process, most probably because they did not need the kind of support that heterosexual women needed and also because usually the methods of insemination were less invasive and less expensive. We also discovered that lesbian couples did not always explain the process anyway, probably because with home conceptions it could appear to breach cultural rules of privacy too much and also sometimes because the couples did not want to worry their parents if, for example, they acquired sperm from an anonymous donor from an Internet site.

> Denise: she told us she was pregnant last year. I went, 'What! bloody hell', I went and I told Donald and he went, 'Bloody hell, how's she managed that?' (301)
>
> Veronica: Presumably she used the – what do they call it – turkey baster. I've never actually really asked, I don't really. (310)
>
> Linda: When I told my dad, I said, 'I've got something to tell you,' and he said, 'Oh, yes.' And I said, 'I'm having a baby,' no, I said, 'I'm pregnant,' and he went, 'How on earth did that happen?' And I said, 'Well, do you want me to tell you?' and he went, 'No, not really' (laughter). (111)
>
> Claudia: I just rang him up one day and said, 'Dad, I need to tell you that Nina's pregnant,' and he was happy, wasn't he?
>
> Nina: He said, 'How did that happen?'
>
> Claudia: Yeah (laughter).
>
> Nina: 'How did that happen?' So we had to go through the whole process. (116)

The predominant response from fathers was one of considerable surprise that their lesbian daughters or their daughter's partner could be pregnant. What we might call the 'How on earth?' response seemed fairly typical. It was not a negative response but one heavily constrained by (now outdated) cultural stereotypes and expectations about the lives of women in same-sex relationships. It appears to combine a slight lack of imagination about alternative mechanics of getting pregnant with an assumption that women who eschew heterosexual relationships also reject motherhood. On the other hand, many of the mothers of lesbian daughters knew very well that their daughters (always) liked and wanted children and so they were less surprised by events.

Where lesbian couples encountered fertility problems, however, the role of mothers became largely the same as the role of mothers of heterosexual daughters. That is to say, where a close relationship was in existence already, then mothers could become immersed in the process. In some cases the parents of lesbian couples already knew the donor and his partner (where it was an informal donation between friends) and so were, in effect, part of the creation of a large network of familial relationships based on different kinds of connections with the donor conceived child. The family networks of the older generation could therefore be quite transformed by the process of donor conception, leading in some cases to connections with the donor's family too. The ripples that went through these families were therefore more muted, with parents often unaware of the process until a pregnancy was announced. Attempting to get pregnant did not consume the older generation in the same way as it did for heterosexual families and, in any case, these parents had faced the possibility that they may not become grandparents at a much earlier stage. They had therefore grieved over their anticipated lack of grandchildren some years previously and thus the prospect of such children being conceived was simply a wonderful bonus.

Phase two: After the birth

a) The families of heterosexual couples

We have described the process of getting pregnant against the odds as a kind of obstacle course which often lasts for years, sometimes as long as a decade. The successful delivery of a child in these circumstances is therefore particularly special. The arrival ends the childlessness of the couple and provides a grandchild to the grandparents but, in the case of donor conception, the child is usually genetically related to only one side of the wider family tree (and of course with embryo donation to neither side). One set of grandparents will therefore be both genetic and legal kin while the other set will be simply legal kin. We discuss in greater detail the significance of genetic connectedness in Chapter 7 but here we focus more broadly on the impact on the wider family of the child's arrival and whether the fact that a child was donor conceived seems to generate specific concerns or disquiet.

One issue that appeared to concern the grandparents was the question of 'belonging'. They were very anxious to ensure that the new arrival belonged in the family and they were ultra-sensitive to anything which might suggest that the child was inappropriately received into the family or treated differently to other grandchildren or the children of other kin. For many grandparents these worries vanished once they saw the infant and the maxim that 'love comes with the child' was one that they adhered to strongly.

> Sheila: I mean when your children arrive, when your grandchildren arrive they're just the same as any of the others. They're there, they're babies, you love them; you form a bond with them. How they are made, I consider to be utterly irrelevant. I mean there are practicalities about that, I don't underestimate that, but they're just the same as the other kids, that's all. (407)
>
> Jacqueline: We do sort of talk about it, but not as much now. I mean I can just see as time goes on, [we] won't be thinking about it that much I'm sure. I wouldn't have thought so, because they become such a little person in their own right, that... she'll be who she is regardless really of, you know, how she came about. (414)

But of course in the case of donor conception the grandparents still had to make an effort, even if it was quite minimal, to conceptualise the new arrival as a fully fledged member of the family. In other words, it required thought and an enthusiastic policy of incorporation; it could not, initially at least, just be taken for granted. Grandparents looked forward to forgetting about the difference between this child and other children in the family.

Where the grandchild had been born through sperm donation, maternal grandparents could also carry forward their concerns about their sons-in-law as they worried that they might not feel secure in their position as father to the child. Where there had been egg donation, maternal grandparents seemed less concerned because they took comfort from the fact that their daughters had carried the pregnancy and given birth. It seemed much easier to forget that a third party had been involved.

> Jacqueline: I said, 'You know, you're going to feel it's yours, because you know, you've got a completely, you go through a completely normal pregnancy you know. Before you know where you are, you'll forget it's not all yours.' (414)

The same kind of comforting narrative could not be offered to infertile men, of course, and so maternal grandparents were sometimes faced with a quandary of how to reassure their sons-in-law that they regarded them as 'true' fathers.

> William: So Jamie's two and a half, or two', nearly two and a half. And I think the main thing we've done with [son-in-law] is to just make sure that he is Jamie's dad as far as we're concerned, isn't he?
> Barbara: Well, he is Jamie's dad.
> William: Yeah, yeah, completely and utterly. (406)

In this exchange between William and Barbara it is possible to see a really genuine concern to reassure their son-in-law about his status as a father, but at the same time their very concentration on this exercise foregrounds their knowledge that he is not a father in the way that most other men become fathers. Their good intentions constantly proclaim the possibility of a shortfall of some kind. To this extent it became clear that grandparents cannot be entirely relaxed about these new forms of relationships brought about by donor conception. None that we interviewed were the slightest bit hostile about these new forms of kinship, but it was clear that they were nonetheless slightly anxious about them and were seeking ways to smooth over possible problems.

To a certain extent the grandparents were also anxious that there might be troubles ahead. One problem was the extent to which children born from donor conception after years of trying to conceive were 'over-loved'. It is not a new discovery to find that different generations have dissimilar approaches to child-rearing, but in cases of children conceived against the odds, grandparents could attribute such differences to the status of the child as an exceptionally precious gift rather than simply generational changes. This was often combined with the fact that the child could be a singleton and that the parents were older than usual and therefore less relaxed about child-rearing.

> Joyce: She's made him very difficult because he's over-loved but then he's a … he's just a very, very, very special child that's been got from huge effort and I don't know. That's why he's so special and why he's over-loved…. My visual picture is of them both if he falls they both rush to pick him up. 'Oh my God he's hurt

himself,' whatever because he's so desperately special to them. Now that obviously has implications.... 404

Jacqueline: Because you notice the difference, um, every little thing, you know. You watch them and you know the danger is you wrap them in cotton wool too much when you've waited so long and that if anything should go wrong... 414

In some of these cases the grandparents could compare the ways in which their other grandchildren were being raised to the over-loving provided to the donor conceived child. While they could obviously understand why the 'special' child was being spoilt, they nonetheless worried about the implications for the future. Of course most grandparents know better than to comment on how their grandchildren are being raised, but in the case of donor conceived children the taboo seems even stricter than usual, leaving grandparents to worry that these children would have problems later in life.

This anticipation of trouble ahead also took the form of a worry that the extraordinary circumstances of the grandchild's conception might incubate psychological or health problems for the future.

William: The complications arise later. When he's a teenager, he'll probably throw it back at everybody around him. (406)

Joanne: [I] just, just hope that all goes well and there's no, no terrible consequences you know some, damage of some kind or other. (408)

Frances: I had a lot of thoughts and, I had – strangely enough, just shortly before she told me she was pregnant, I'd heard on the radio an interview with someone who had been donor conceived, a girl – a woman, who was in her twenties, who was very, very bitter... about the fact that she didn't have background for half of herself. She said she didn't know who she was and so bitter. So... that upset me a bit because I, you know, I wouldn't want that to happen to [my grandchildren]. (413)

These kinds of uncertainties, and also qualms about the introduction of different and unknown gene pools which we discuss in Chapter 7, suggest yet again that no matter how welcomed the donor conceived child is into the wider family, he or she comes accompanied with vague niggling worries about how things will work out in future.

We do not suggest that these kinds of concerns only appear in circumstances of donor conception, but it is important to acknowledge that such fears do circulate even where the child is warmly received. In part these kinds of worries are an inevitable adjunct to any form of innovation in the shaping of contemporary kinship. These grandparents (and also aunts and uncles, siblings and cousins) had no direct experience of alternative families, except where there might have been an adoption in the past. Thus they were susceptible to negative narratives, such as the one noted above of the embittered donor conceived woman heard on the radio. They might carry forward understandings about failed and difficult adoptions, or they may have heard vague media stories of sperm donors passing on disabling conditions.

> Cathryn: [My mother] still had a lot of... very dated ideas about well, you know, 'What if she's a criminal? You know, then you've got criminal genes in your family.' (201)

b) The families of lesbian couples

We suggest above that, except in cases of infertility, the parents of lesbian couples were not necessarily hugely involved in the story of the conception. Moreover, once the child was born they were not, unlike the families of heterosexual couples, in a position to 'forget' about the donor conception and carry on as nearly 'normal'. These grandparents were faced with a very different family structure and some struggled with this, especially if they had never really accepted the sexual orientation of their daughter. They were also often very worried about the future.

A crucial factor in how these grandparents reacted seemed to relate to who the birth mother of the grandchild was because the parents of birth mothers often felt far more secure and connected than the parents of the non-genetic mother. This insecurity could be related to a number of factors; for example, whether or not the couple had a civil partnership, whether both mothers appeared on the birth certificate, whether the non-genetic mother had adopted the child, whether or not they liked and trusted the birth mother and also whether they approved of the whole arrangement in the first place. This dynamic was completely unique to the parents of lesbian couples, of course, and the parents of heterosexual couples seemed not to give a moment's consideration to whether they should welcome the child or whether they could lose contact with their grandchildren.

This insecurity felt by some of the grandparents was completely understandable given the complexities of lesbian donor conception. Some grandchildren were born from anonymously donated sperm bought from the Internet and if there was no civil partnership then non-genetic grandparents could not have any legal standing at all. In cases where there was informal donation from a known donor then the parents of the donor would be, in law, the 'real' grandparents and not the parents of the non-genetic mother. Moreover, the exact status of the non-genetic mother has changed considerably over the last decade, leaving a general sense of confusion and insecurity which only legal adoption by the non-genetic mother was able, at one point, to resolve.

> Betty: But, you know, at first, when he was little, I used to think, 'Oh, (long pause), what would I do if Kirsty ever took him off us?' you know. I did used to think that. But as I say, as the years have gone on – And I mean, she's said, 'Whatever happens, even now, you know, even though Mary's adopted him,' she said, 'I'd never, if me and Mary split up, I'd never ever take [grandson] away from you. He'd always be part of your life.' (314)

Betty and her husband, Richard, were both clear that the adoption process had made them feel more secure even though they insisted that they had regarded their grandson as 'theirs' from the moment of his birth.

But not all non-genetic grandparents felt this degree of automatic connection because they felt that there was no family connection.

> Nancy: [My daughter's partner] is the birth mother right. Which kind of saddened me a little bit because I had kind of hoped that we would have something of our family, maybe even an embryo, an egg, something. (302)

One other set of non-genetic grandparents we interviewed were faced with a situation in which their daughter's partner had removed their grandchild altogether and were refusing to let them see him. She also tried to stop their daughter seeing her son and the whole matter ended up in court.

> Anita: I actually said...that she'd got the ability to break our daughter's heart by taking [grandson] if something happened between them. I actually said this to her and she wrote to me a letter, a very sweet letter...saying that she would never do that even if they split up she would never do that cause...the baby would love [our daughter]. But look what happened. Exactly as I forecast. But I didn't have any problem with them having a baby together personally. (306)

This lack of connection could give rise to anxiety for non-genetic kin but the flipside of this coin was that non-genetic kin could also just ignore the child and fail to acknowledge his or her existence as a member of the wider family. This might mean that although non-genetic grandparents acknowledged the child, non-genetic uncles or aunts might not. The child could be seen as 'none of their business' or as a bit of an embarrassment. In one case the father of one of the lesbian mothers we interviewed had remarried a younger woman and so had children who were teenagers when his grandchild was due to be born. His reaction was to insist that his children were not told about the child, at least not for the time being, thus potentially cutting off one part of his family from the other.

The biggest anxiety that grandparents seemed to encounter was, however, the fear of discrimination both against the couple and potentially against their grandchildren. The feeling was that in having children the couple were making their 'difference' more visible, which could invite demonstrations of hostility. In addition, it was thought that the children themselves would encounter bullying at school once it was known that they came from non-traditional families.

> Nancy: My husband was a little bit more reserved, [because] he really did know what he was going to encounter with this. I don't know, he just saw it in a different light.
> Interviewer: How do you mean?
> Nancy: Well in the bigotry of the world, um, he worried about it. Whereas I put it aside and didn't want to think about that.

I wanted to see the happy part. I didn't want to see anything
else. I didn't want to see the ugly. Whereas he was worried about
the ugly part you know. (302)

Theresa: Then you have bullying. And how does a child cope with
that? They don't realise all these things you know. So it's very
difficult sometimes yeah. (303)

These anxious grandparents still seemed to long for heterosexual
daughters because, in their view, their lesbian daughters had chosen a
difficult path and it was quite likely that they would face hard times.
They sometimes found that it was hard to tell acquaintances and
even friends that they had become grandparents because they did
not want to explain the details of conception and parentage to people who might be unreceptive or shocked. These grandparents were
unhappy because they thought the 'world' was not ready for alternative family forms and they wanted to avoid unpleasantness. But there
were equal numbers of grandparents who seemed to think that the
world had changed sufficiently to accommodate lesbian mothers.

Judith: Yeah it really depends, one of the things that, you know has
come up is the fact that [my daughter's] older sister, she's almost
two years older, has been married for ten years and she and her
husband chose not to have children and so it's like, 'Oh well
your heterosexual daughter doesn't have a child and your gay
daughter does' and so it's kind of, you know, how the world has
changed in many respects and the acceptance that this is quite
normal. (304)

These differences of perception may have been linked to a number
of factors but important among them was clearly location because
grandparents living in parts of cosmopolitan London were rather
relaxed about such matters, while those living abroad or in more traditional and/or small neighbourhoods were much more worried. And
it was clear that even those who were at the most relaxed end of the
continuum had reservations about telling everyone they knew about
the full facts of their grandchild's circumstances.

The birth of a grandchild to lesbian parents could also have
the effect of 'healing' strained family relationships. A focus on
a grandchild, no matter how conceived, could obliterate other

considerations which suddenly seemed to become less significant. The child could also become a bridge which connected both sides of the family and this connection could even extend to include known donors and their partners. We explore this kind of healing through one particular case, that of Gemma and Sasha. Gemma's mother was a social worker who lived in the North of England while Sasha's mother was a Conservative councillor living on the south coast. The two sides of the family could not have been more different, with one side being totally at ease with their daughter's sexuality and decision to have a child, and the other side uncomprehending, almost verging on hostile at first.

> Gemma: And I was down there and I said something about having kids and your mum said, 'I don't think people like you should have kids.' But she was so, she was just, it was genuine ignorance wasn't it? She didn't know any other gay couples, she didn't really know, I don't know if it was just a kneejerk reaction. (114)

By comparison, Gemma's mother was entirely happy with the situation:

> Gemma: My mum thinks it's a marvellous idea to have kids with another woman, because they're so much better than men at looking after kids, and being helped in the house and, she thinks from a pragmatic point of view, it's a much better idea [than] having kids than in straight relationships. And she does say if she had her time again [she would do it with a woman] (laughs).

However, on the birth of their first daughter Sasha's mother was transformed and became besotted with her (and also the subsequent) granddaughter.

> Gemma: I think, well it's the same with anyone who's prejudiced isn't it. I think she still does hold some of her prejudices doesn't she, but she kind of makes exceptions for [us].
> Sasha: Yes. I don't think, I mean she's gone from being someone who would never have told any of her friends, to telling everyone and whenever we went home with either of the children, she'd

invite all her friends round to have these grandchildren, this is my grandchild you know and get people really involved in it. But now she's got friends who've got gay children so she's had more of a, kind of exposure if you like.

...

Sasha: And also, I mean we've been together for what 17 years, she's had quite a long time to get her head round it.

Gemma: And things have changed, everyone's changed I think....

Sasha: Yes and I think the fact I'm out at work and work knows and we've had our civil partnership and we've had our commitment ceremony. My dad had a heart attack and I think that was a real wake up call to her, that actually, because her attitude after that changed massively.

Gemma: That was, that was about three or four years after we met wasn't it.

Sasha: Yes, because I think she suddenly thought, life is too short to be bitter about things.

The story of Sasha's mother is archetypal in that it documents how the ripples through families can operate, sometimes taking years, and sometimes combining with other significant events over time (e.g. a heart attack) to create a huge change in both attitudes and relationships. Gemma and Sasha were wise enough to realise that Sasha's mother had not let go of all her prejudices but they were genuinely pleased about how far she had moved. They both also acknowledge that it was harder for her than it was for Gemma's mother because Gemma was the birth mother to both children which meant that Sasha's mother did not have a genetic link with the children. Sasha's parents' upbringings were also very conventional and, as Sasha pointed out in the interview, when she first came out (some 17 years or more previously) probably the only other gay person they would have met might have been a hairdresser, in other words someone who fitted a particular stereotype and who was also situated at a great distance from them both socially and professionally. Thus gay people went from being quite 'other' to becoming very close members of their family and they needed time to accommodate to the seismic shift.

Conclusion

The reactions of wider family to donor conception appear to vary considerably in cases where the parents of the donor conceived children are a heterosexual couple compared with when they are a same-sex couple. For heterosexual couples the wider family, particularly grandparents, become crucial in providing support through the process of conception but after a child is born, the whole family tries to return to near 'normal', which is to say that, for grandparents, life goes on largely as 'it should do' and the blip of infertility is rendered a distant albeit painful memory. This does not mean that life goes on entirely smoothly (see Chapters 4 and 5) but order is restored to a large extent. In contrast, for lesbian couples the wider family is usually held at arm's length during the conception process and it is after the birth of a child that serious adjustments have to begin. If these grandparents (and other relatives) want to have a relationship with the new grandchild then bridges have to be built and the new family unit has to be acknowledged. We came across only two cases where parents remained implacable. The first was where the grandparents refused to acknowledge the new family and insisted on telling all other relatives and friends that their daughter had a boyfriend who had fathered her child. The second case involved one of the older lesbians we interviewed whose children were almost grown up. Her parents refused to acknowledge her son because she was not his birth mother, and also failed to include her daughter in bequests even though she was her birth mother. In this case Susan no longer regarded her parents as kin. It is, of course, more than likely that this kind of denial happens more frequently than we found in our study and it is also possible that even more grandparents deny all knowledge of grandchildren born to lesbian mothers. However, the dominant story that we heard was the one where the birth of a child led to a warming of cool relationships, and sometimes even a complete transformation.

Our interviews with grandparents and also the questions we asked parents about their wider families revealed the extent to which family networks are crucially significant where there is donor conception. The response of grandparents could make a great difference to whether or not parents could create a proper sense of belonging to a family for their children. It also seemed to be very important to parents that their own parents accepted their children and did not treat them at all differently from other sets of grandchildren. Grandparents themselves felt that they had no right to interfere in the decisions of their adult children (Nordqvist and Smart, forthcoming 2014) but this does not mean that the parents did not need their support. In the next two chapters we explore precisely how these delicate intergenerational relationships work in relation to the complex issues of telling children and also the wider world about the nature of their conception. The whole process of 'telling', or not 'telling' wider kin, let alone wider social networks, had direct impact on grandparents, some of whom found more modern ideas of transparency rather difficult. In later chapters too, grandparents will reappear as key actors in how the donor is perceived and also in how to manage knowledge about genetic difference.

4
Keeping It Close: Sensitivities and Secrecy

This chapter explores how donor conception can give rise to secrets and sensitivities in families. Secrecy has a long history in the context of donor conception (Haimes, 1992; Kirkman, 2005) and recent studies suggest that it remains an important feature of the life of families of donor conceived children. For example, Readings *et al.* (2011), Grace and Daniels (2007), Murray and Golombok (2003) and MacCallum (2009), who draw on heterosexual clinic-based samples, indicate that a significant proportion of parents of embryo-, egg- and sperm-donor conceived babies intend never to disclose the details of their conception. MacCallum (2009) found that 43 per cent of mothers and 56 per cent of fathers of embryo conceived children were intending to keep the facts around the embryo donation a secret. Studies focusing on donor insemination (Grace and Daniels, 2007) and egg donation (Murray and Golombok, 2003) have also found that a high proportion of parents intend never to reveal the genetically 'true' background of their children (see also Appleby *et al.*, 2012).

Secrecy and discretion was also a strong theme emerging in the interviews that we conducted, and this suggests that concealment continues to play an important role in families of donor conceived children and how parents perceive and manage information about donor conception. In this chapter we explore how donor conception can be seen as so sensitive that some families decide to keep the information to themselves, or to tell only a select few. We address how it becomes something that families want to, or feel the need to, manage discreetly and why it is that people decide that it is information that is better kept private. We also explore how secrets start to expand in families and how they become something that family members 'manage' as part of relating to one another. Finally, we investigate how secrets impact on the lives of these families and also their visions of the future.

It is important to emphasise that the secrets that were guarded in these families could take a number of different forms. Usually, in heterosexual families, the secret focused on the use of a donor. However, in lesbian families, the secret could revolve around the same-sex relationship as well as the donation. Although secrets emerged for different reasons, there was a common thread in these stories and families, which was the desire to keep information about the family hidden. To clarify all these different elements the chapter is divided into four sections. First, we investigate how families perceive reproductive donation in a way that leads them to decide to keep some information private. In the second section, we go on to explore how families keep information from spreading and the different strategies that families use to keep information to themselves. Third, we look at how information about donor conception becomes guarded and how, as a consequence, it acquires a powerful potency, such that letting go is perceived as risky and dangerous. In the final section we investigate how parents and grandparents perceive the future when the donation has been kept a secret.

Sensitive information and maximum discretion

Sensitivities to donor conception started to grow for a variety of reasons in the families who took part in our study. Many parents felt reluctant to share information because they believed that their child should be in charge of the process once they were old enough. The parents did not see the information as rightfully theirs to share. This idea was grounded in a belief that the information about donor conception concerned, first and foremost, the donor conceived child. For some parents, such as the lesbian couple Amber and Heather, this meant that they refused to share information about their conception process with anyone before their son was old enough to be told.

> Amber: What we say [when people ask] is that well, 'No, I appreciate you want to know but we think it's really important that [our son] is the first person to know that.'
> Heather: So it's a family decision that we don't tell anybody. (105)

Both maternal grandmothers had been curious and asked about how their grandson had been conceived, but the couple believed strongly that the means of conception was only their son's concern:

> Amber: It's whose business it is, and it's [our son's] business. Why is it in any way your mum's business or my mum's business? What difference would it make to my mum's life if she knew how we'd conceived him?... It's not relevant to that relationship.

Another example emerged in our interview with grandmother Shirley, who had a grandson through egg donation. Her daughter had explained to her that it was up to the boy to decide when and how the information should be shared:

> Shirley: [My daughter says] it isn't fair to tell everyone. That's up to [my grandson], who [he] wants to know and when he get[s] to be older. (409)

Clearly, the daughter had told her own mother about the son's genetic donor, but the boy's parents were otherwise very restrictive about sharing information more widely.

Ideas about information ownership underpinning these two stories are grounded in cultural beliefs about identity and genetic family origins, on the one hand, and convictions about a right to privacy, on the other. As we discussed in Chapter 1, in the Euro-American context a person's identity is conceptually linked with his or her genetic family (Strathern, 1992; Edwards, 2000). It might be said that the cultural notion of personal identity is *co-constituted* with genetic kinship. This means that genetic family background is understood to carry information about personal background and identity and that a person's kin connections are seen to provide knowledge about the person. When individuals learn something about their genetic family background, they are perceived to learn something about themselves. They have learnt something that is understood to constitute their identity. Because information about donor conception is seen as constitutive of the identity of the donor conceived person, such information is also recognised to be profoundly personal, and it thereby becomes an issue of privacy. Although privacy remains notoriously difficult to define (Inness, 1992) it holds significant social currency and there is a widespread legal and social notion of a 'right' to privacy (Richards, 2008). As with any deeply personal information, there is a perception that a person has the right to decide for themselves with whom to share it and from whom to withhold it. These parents' decision to keep information from leaking out is situated in these cultural ideas about identity, kinship, personhood, privacy and ownership.

There are also moral undertones embedded in these accounts. Shirley noted, for example, that it would be unfair on her grandson to share the information without his consent. Equally, Amber and Heather's account suggested that they perceived this to be the only morally right way of managing the information. These parents therefore felt that they were doing the right thing by their child in keeping the information as confidential as possible.

In addition to these ideas on privacy we found that some parents worried that others would react with disapproval. They feared that people would condemn donor conception as a practice, and would start treating them and their child negatively. Parents could not, of course, be sure of what the reaction would be, but the fear itself was a powerful disincentive to disclosure. Clive and Stephanie had a son through egg donation. They both felt worried about being open about having used a donor.

> Clive: You can stand the openness and be open with everybody so they all know and that's fine when people are happy with it, with that piece of information .... I guess my concern is when people have their own opinions and when they find out and then they maybe look at us differently or look at [our son] differently and treat him differently ... cause you know people are I guess, some people would say 'Yeah that's great' and other people when they haven't gone through that experience will think, 'Well you know it wasn't meant to be, so therefore why have you gone down that route?' (214)

Although there may be a broad acceptance of donor conception in the UK (as witnessed by the provision of such services in the NHS), this permissiveness may not apply to the local context of specific families of donor conceived children. Clive and Stephanie were both Christians and active members in their local church, and their faith and faith group were an important part of their personal life. They were, however, not sure that everyone in the community would approve of their route to parenthood. Clive's notion that some might react by saying 'It was not meant to be' can be understood in this religious context as Clive and Stephanie feared that others might see infertility treatment and egg donation as acting against God's will. In many religious contexts reproductive technologies and assisted donor conception remain widely disapproved of and the use of them therefore deeply stigmatised (e.g. Culley and Hudson, 2006; Fenton, 2006; Inhorn, 2007). Parents such as Clive and Stephanie were unsure of what would come of openness and therefore chose to remain secretive.

It was not only parents in religious communities who feared that others would react with disapproval. Donor conception was also felt to be a socially and culturally contentious issue in other networks and families, thus making disclosure a fraught and uncertain process for most parents. What made disclosure appear so risky for many parents was not only the thought that they themselves could stand to lose important relationships and face disapproval, but that this could happen to their child. Fiona and her husband, Brian, had a daughter through egg donation. They kept the conception completely secret from family and friends for the first 18 months of their daughter's life, but eventually decided that they wanted to be more open. Fiona talks about the time before they started telling, and how risky the prospect of openness seemed to her then:

> Fiona: The biggest worry I had for when we were starting to tell, [was] that anybody would reject [our daughter] .... It's a real visceral thing, isn't it? It's a real sort of gut reaction thing, you know, to protect your child and that was my ... They could have said and done anything to me, called me you know, the biggest freak under the sun and it wouldn't have, I couldn't have cared less. But the thought that anybody might say 'Oh well, she's not part of our family then is she?' ... Even though I know that that would never have happened, 'cause I know my family, I was still worried you know. (204)

The prospect that a child could be rejected by the family was truly worrying and so parents had to balance the possible risks before disclosing the information. Families and children's lives are linked to the lives of family networks, and these relationships are an important part of personal life (Bengtson *et al.*, 2002). These networks play a vital role and they cannot easily be abandoned or ignored if their response is unfavourable or judgemental (Smart 2007). This meant that the threat that a grandparent, for example, might not accept the child as a grandchild was experienced as very serious and could propel parents into keeping the donation a secret. Whereas Fiona and Brian eventually decided to take the risk and open up, for other parents the balance went the other way. Danielle and Christina, for example, who used both donated sperm and eggs for the conception of a second child, found it necessary to keep the information about the donor eggs from the wider family:

> Danielle: I do not intend to tell my family that he's not my biological child. . . . I'm not telling my family because I don't know how they would feel about it and whether they would then regard the child as less of a, you know, family member maybe. (106)

Imparting information about donor conception was thus experienced as having a very powerful potential to alter relationships. This perceived potency relates to cultural ideas about the meaning of kinship and how knowledge about genetic kin has the power, in an instant, to change relationships. Marilyn Strathern (1999) has written about the particular kind of knowledge that comes with genetic kinship connections/disconnections, suggesting that information about kinship connections has the power to transform relationships:

> [W]e shall not understand. . . people's reluctance, or their desire to not-know, or anxieties about where information will lead, unless we realise that kinship knowledge has certain built-in effects.
>
> (Strathern, 1999:69)

Once we understand these built-in effects, we can better appreciate that disclosure about genetic disconnectedness was for some a very risky prospect, as they feared that relationships would alter as a consequence.

In our study, it was not uncommon for the grandparents of the donor conceived child to be the ones most against the information spreading to the wider family. Lea and Joshua had both experienced infertility, and had eventually conceived a daughter using IVF and sperm donation. While the couple wanted to share this information quite openly, Lea's mother was less keen. Lea explained her mother's viewpoint:

> Lea: I'm kind of perceived as the successful one among my cousins, they're all kind of a bit odd. So everyone says, 'Oh, she's done well and she's got friends and she's kind of normal'. And my mum said, 'Oh, you know, if they found out you had some serious problems [with infertility] they'll be actually happy about it'. And said, 'Why should they talk badly about you? Why should we give them any reasons to talk about it?' So that's a bit of a dynamic, which I don't really care about one bit. (206)

A number of processes are at work in this quotation. Although this is a short account, it provides great insight into family relationships, and how donor conception becomes part of these relationships. It appears that Lea was part of a family which, on her mother's side, was prone to discussing and judging the relative successes (or failures) of sons, daughters and cousins. Clearly a certain amount of competitiveness shaped these relationships. It would seem that Lea, who according to her mother was seen as the 'successful one', was a source of pride to her mother, and this could lead to jealousy among other members of the family. The grandmother appears to suspect that the failure to conceive, and so the need to use IVF and donor sperm, meant that Lea might slip down the cousin hierarchy in the eyes of the relatives. In the same way that other parents hesitated to share news about donor conception because they feared that relatives might receive it unfavourably, it was clear that well-nurtured reputations could also be at stake in some families. So a grandparent could decide to guard the information as a way of keeping up a façade to more distant relatives.

We found another example of a similar dynamic in our interview with Sheryl. She was a single mother of a donor conceived child, Jennifer, who she had had in the context of a previous relationship with Penny. Sheryl's parents strongly disapproved of the circumstances of their grandchild's birth. They disliked the fact that Sheryl was a lesbian and could not accept the idea of the donor conception. They insisted on keeping both the relationship and the donation a secret from the wider family who Sheryl described as 'very, very traditional'. It would appear they felt strongly that the news that their daughter was a lesbian must not be known because they had also lied to their relatives, telling them that little Jennifer was conceived as the result of a heterosexual alliance. They had even given the imaginary father a name and a career. Sheryl became aware of the extent of her mother's disapproval as she got talking to a friend of her mother's at work:

> Sheryl: I've just started this job and there's a lady that actually works on my team who is a friend of my mum's and we've only just realised this and we had this brief discussion, she said, 'Oh yeah I didn't know [name] was your mum,' and then she kind of turned around and said, 'Oh yeah you're never really talked about are you? Your mum's always talking about your brother but she never talks about you.' So obviously that's hit home to me, obviously I'm just kind of this black sheep and I don't even get mentioned. (115)

Sheryl's family situation had become more complex over time. When Jennifer was two, Sheryl took her and moved to be near her own parents, and as a consequence the couple relationship broke down. Her ex-partner, Penny, met a new woman and went on to have another child by the same donor. This meant that Jennifer had a (half) sister. Jennifer and her sister were still young, but Penny kept in touch and Jennifer knew about her baby sister. The grandparents had also been told about the baby but found the idea of talking to their granddaughter about it abhorrent and tried to discourage her from having contact.

> Sheryl: [When I told my parents about the baby they] were just like, 'Well that's ridiculous and it's nothing to do with you and you don't want Jennifer getting involved 'cause it's going to mess her up and it's going to affect her later on in life.'

It might be assumed that a parent could simply ignore or bypass the grandparents' request to keep things secret but this would underestimate the importance of family relationships and embeddedness in wider kin networks. Intergenerational relationships can be vital in personal life, and this is particularly so at the point at which a new generation is born into the family (Bengtson *et al.*, 2002). A parent might not be able to share the information freely with other relatives without risking damaging their relationship with their own parents, and with that, their child's relationship with their grandparent. In Sheryl's case, the situation was particularly difficult because Sheryl was a single mother on a low income and lived in a housing association flat. She relied heavily on her own mother for childcare and support. It is therefore possible to see that an open confrontation with her parents, with the potential outcome of support being withdrawn, may have had very difficult consequences for Sheryl and Jennifer. The issue of donor conception could be very delicate, especially in cases where going against decisions to keep things secret would mean challenging forceful and long-standing structures of power in families (Zerubavel, 2006; Nippert-Eng, 2010).

These accounts thus show how decisions about secrecy are embedded in already existing family relationships that have developed over time (Finch and Mason, 1993). Many parents (as well as grandparents) experienced sharing information within the family against the wishes of another family member as potentially damaging important relationships. Thus many families balanced their own desires for more openness with their and their children's need for these important relationships to continue.

Managing sensitivities

It was very difficult for couples and family members to keep information about infertility treatment and donor conception completely hidden from view. Often, it was not an option to say nothing at all because, as we discussed in Chapter 3, mothers who underwent treatment often felt the need to share the burden with at least one close relative, usually a person they could really trust. To keep the treatment and subsequent donor conception entirely to themselves was therefore often not an option. Erin, for example, initially went through a series of unsuccessful IVF treatment cycles which caused her difficulties over a number of years.

> Erin: I just didn't feel like I could talk to people, many people, about it so I probably...I mean no more than a handful, I mean a small handful, like three people I'd say. I talked to my mum, I talked to one of my closest friends who has also gone through IVF treatment and probably maybe one, maybe two other people, but not in such depth.... Simply because I got in such a state that you know it was kind of impossible for them to [not] realise that something was going on and I just had to talk to somebody about it. (217)

In the context of lesbian donation, the birth of a child also made it very difficult to hide a lesbian relationship, both for the couple as well as for relatives. A child needed to be explained, and so brought the couple relationship into the open (Almack, 2007). So families often had to balance wanting to keep things secret but finding that actually doing so was very difficult. Some parents and grandparents in our study resolved this tension by telling a partial truth about their family. This was, for example, illustrated in Clive and Stephanie's account. Clive mentioned telling a cousin about the difficulties that they had experienced conceiving, but it emerged that he had not told the whole truth.

> Clive: The only other family [than my parents] I've told is [my second cousin].
> Stephanie: What have you told him?
> Clive: I've told him something.
> Stephanie: You haven't told him about donor eggs have you?...I don't think you told him about donor eggs, [but] I'm sure he knew that we were having trouble....(214)

It was common for the heterosexual couples to choose to disclose details about having had problems conceiving and having been through infertility treatment, but without also mentioning having used a donor. Another example of this was found in our interview with Elizabeth and Adrian; only here it was Elizabeth's mother who insisted on not sharing information about the donation. That side of the family had, however, been told that the child was a 'fertility baby':

> Petra: So on your mum's side, her brothers and sisters, [they] haven't been told [about the donation]?
> Elizabeth: Yeah, not that I'm aware of.... [But] I think they know he's a fertility baby. My gran definitely knows he's a fertility baby.
> Adrian: But I think it would be your mum who would be embarrassed for some reason about telling them. (221)

It was also common for family members of lesbian couples to reveal a partial truth about the birth of a child. In our study, it was typically the grandparents who were unwilling to mention their daughter's sexuality. Linda's father had received the news of Linda's relationship with Dawn, and also her pregnancy, with disquiet. At first, he had asked her not to tell her younger half-siblings. But keeping quiet about a new relationship and the arrival of a child had not been easy, especially as the pregnancy started to show, and eventually the siblings had been told. However, Linda was made aware that her father felt ongoing discomfort about the situation as she ran into an old family friend one day:

> Linda: One day shortly after [our son] was born, we were in Selfridges, in [city], and we bumped into this woman who was a friend of the family for years and years and I said, 'Hello, how are you?' And she said, 'Oh, hi,' and I said, 'This is my son and this is my partner, Dawn,' and she said, 'That explains everything,' and I said, 'Oh right.' She said she'd run into my dad, my dad had said, 'Linda's having a baby', and this woman had said, 'Oh, who's the father?' and Dad said, 'There is no father.' So he would rather that I'd had a one-night stand and got pregnant than Dad actually tell her I'm in a relationship with a woman, and, you know, ... I was quite sad about that, but, you know, that's just my dad. (111)

Clearly, this was hurtful for Linda, who drew the conclusion that her father preferred not to mention her relationship. Many similar stories emerged in our interviews about lesbian donation. Amber and Heather, for example, mentioned that Amber's father, who lived abroad, would introduce Amber to his friends only if she came to visit on her own, and never if the couple travelled together. Nancy, a grandmother, told us that both she and her husband took enormous pleasure in their grandchildren, but did not mention to neighbours that their daughter was a lesbian. They also lived abroad, and the geographical distance made it easier to reveal only a portion of the truth. This strategy was more fraught for someone in Linda's situation because the family lived geographically close by and the truth would almost inevitably seep out.

The families also tried to resolve not wanting to share information too widely and having to explain themselves, by controlling the flow of information. However, because grandparents often already knew the details they could in turn be requested to keep the information to themselves:

> Jennifer (with Robert): We'd had a discussion with [our parents] early on to say, you know, we'd appreciate it if you don't discuss this with... [W]e had said to them what we felt that, you know, it was the kids' information. And so really, you know, the kids should be in charge of who knows eventually. (210)
>
> Clive (with Stephanie): [We have told our parents] but that's where it finishes. (214)

This finding was echoed in our interviews with grandparents who spoke of not being 'allowed' to share the information that was imparted to them. For example, Sally spoke of her daughter who struggled with infertility and who endured infertility exploration and treatment for ten years before successful conception. For the first five years, the daughter's only confidant was her mother, who was asked to keep the information to herself:

> Sally: Although I knew all about it, she didn't want other people to know. She didn't want anybody else, no one in the family to know. (411)

To keep these boundaries in place was, however, not necessarily an easy task as it was impossible to know if others honoured the request to not talk about the donation. For example, Shirley's daughter and her husband were very protective of what they perceived to be their son's right to be in charge of the information, and were very cautious about who they told. They had told both of their mothers and both of her brothers, but they had chosen not to tell the husband's sister as they feared she would gossip. Shirley's daughter had expected her brothers to keep the information to themselves, but one brother had told his wife:

> Shirley: [My daughter said] 'I told [my brother] and he's told [his wife].' She didn't like that, I could tell from her tone. (409)

The families who wanted to keep information a secret but had confided in a select few had to contend with the risk of their secrets leaking out.

These risks were especially prominent in some families where the parents had reason to suspect that the secret might not be very safe. This issue was addressed with some force in our interview with Robyn and Malinda. Both women were on a low income, and this had prevented them from accessing sperm donor treatment in a clinic (Nordqvist, 2011a). Instead, they tried to conceive in an informal arrangement. Finding a suitable donor proved very difficult, however, and after some unsuccessful attempts, Robyn's mother suggested that they approach an old friend of the family. The man was married and had no children of his own. He agreed but on the condition that his wife, who had always wanted to have children by him, never found out about his contribution. He feared that the arrangement could potentially break up his marriage; it therefore seemed extremely important that it remained a secret. Robyn and Malinda had run out of options and were extremely grateful to the man who might enable them to have a child, and so decided to go ahead. Robyn conceived, and at the time of the interview the daughter was two years old. Although the donor remained a friend of the family and knew the little girl, his identity as her donor was going to be kept secret from her and everyone else. This was the only case in our study in which the parents were planning to keep information about the donation from the child herself. The 'official' story was that the donor had been a lodger who had stayed with the grandmother for a short spell. But the parents were not the only ones who knew the truth. Robyn's mother, the child's grandmother, had known from the beginning and this caused the couple some concern:

Robyn: I spoke to [my mother] before I [asked] the donor [if he would donate] and said – because my mum can be a bit of a blabber mouth and my biggest fear was, when [our daughter] gets older and she's like, 'Nanny tell me, nanny tell me,' is my mum going to still be strong and stick to the story? So that was my concern. So I sat down with her first and foremost and spoke to her and said, 'You know you can't break her heart and you can't break mine and you know these are the risks that this donor is taking for me to do this and you've got to, you've got to keep this secret.' And it wasn't until she got how important it was, that I went and spoke to the donor.

Malinda: How important it is to him as well, isn't it? And then you did reiterate it when she was born.

Robyn: Yes and I think I did a couple of months ago as well and I will continue to do so. (117)

Although Robyn had got her mother to promise never to reveal the secret before she went ahead with the donation, it appears that she still felt uncertain that she could trust her not to do so. She therefore had to work at keeping the donation a secret but they also lived with the ongoing risk that it would be revealed.

Pandora's box

The donation gradually acquired a powerful potency in the families who kept information hidden because, over time, it grew into a sensitive and delicate matter. The problem that developed in these families can be understood as something of a Pandora's box; the families worked hard to keep the lid on the box and to stop information from leaking out. This was, for example, illustrated in our interview with Shirley. Shirley lived in a small village, and her daughter, son-in-law and donor conceived grandson lived up the road from her. On meeting Shirley at the train station on arrival, she explained with some urgency that she would not introduce the interviewer, or explain her reason for visiting, if they happened to run into anyone. The following extract is from our field notes:

As we walked from the station to her car she said, 'Petra, I should tell you that this is such a small village and if we meet anyone, I will introduce you as a friend but I won't mention the donor thing. I might mention the IVF but I won't mention the donor thing because this is such a small village and no one knows about the donor.' (409)

It was clear that Shirley took a risk when taking part in the study, as it might have meant that information was unveiled. In the interview, she spoke about her daughter's wish to keep the donation secret and Shirley said that she had not told her own friends about it. She talked about one friend in particular, Doris, who she was close to and who she was going to meet later that day, but who did not know about the donation:

> Shirley: I have a very, very close, dear friend, Doris, I normally see her today and we've got a little bit of a mix-up. And I wouldn't be a bit surprised if she turned up. But Doris would be the very last person [I would tell]. I love her to pieces; she is a wonderful, wonderful friend, but she is so open. She would just tell – not gossiping, not a gossip, just very open and she would say, 'Did you know [Shirley's grandson] was donor conceived? Did you? Well, isn't that lovely?' ... She would tell everyone. The whole world and his wife would know (laughter) .... And this morning I've had to say to Doris, because she's actually rung this morning, 'I'm picking a friend up from the station.' You see, now, when I see her she'll want to know who this friend was and I'm thinking, what can I say to Doris (laughter)? So I'm going to be a bit vague. She doesn't play bridge, Doris, so she doesn't know my friends at the bridge club so I'm going to tell a little white lie which I don't like doing, but I'm just going to vaguely say, 'Oh, she's from the bridge club,' and change the subject. (laughter)

It would appear that the interview itself brought out some of the issues that Shirley had to manage because of the secrecy. This was most likely a very unusual event in Shirley's life, but it nevertheless highlighted how carefully this grandmother worked to protect her daughter's secret. It also shows the potency that the information had acquired over time. It had grown into something that became a Pandora's box in the family and this grandmother struggled to hold the lid in place.

Opening the lid of this Pandora's box of donor conception was perceived as a risky and dangerous prospect. The imagined risks were manifold, and different for different families. In Shirley's case, the potential danger was the perceived loss of the grandson's right to privacy, and perhaps also her daughter's confidence. Robyn and Malinda, who worked to keep their donor's identity secret, imagined that disclosure would have disastrous consequences both for them and for the donor. Clive and Stephanie imagined risking the support of their religious community, Danielle worried that her non-genetic child would not be welcomed as part of the family and Sheryl was concerned that her parents would stop supporting her. These perceived dangers would be unleashed irreversibly if the lid on this Pandora's box was removed.

To understand the fear of this risk we need to situate donor conception, and the information contained within it, in a cultural context of kinship thinking. Following Strathern (1999:79) the Euro-American idea of biological ties 'has the character of a constitutive finality that cannot be modified, that once known cannot be laid aside'. This means that once information about donor conception is 'out of the box' the effects are immediate; new knowledge about relationships has already been formed. Smart (2011:550) has previously noted that 'reproductive secrets in families have the power to be disruptive and dangerous because, once revealed, they will always alter relationships'. These families do not have the option of taking back the information if the consequences of disclosure are as disastrous as they imagine. For example, Danielle could not 'undo' telling her family about using an egg donor if they reacted by excluding the child from the family. This is why information about the donation could over time acquire an almost volatile and explosive potential to disrupt and disturb and also why it came to be treated as such a delicate matter in many families.

A twisting tale: Imagining the future

In most of the families we spoke to, it seemed that an initial commitment to secrecy could change over time. It was clear that the secret was likely to be revealed sooner or later. Often, this was because the parents were planning to tell their children that they were donor conceived from a young age anyway (we discuss this further in

Chapter 5). Sally was a grandmother of an embryo donation child. Her daughter had struggled for a decade with infertility, undergoing different treatment regimes. They had always been, and still were, very secretive about the child's genetic origins. The daughter was, however, adamant that the boy should know, and she had already started telling him when he was two years old.

> Sally: Secrets are not a good idea... especially as actually in the end, if [my grandson] chooses to stand on the rooftop and shout it, he's going to, isn't he?... And [my daughter] will not tell him 'It's going to be a secret.' She said, 'I'm not going to tell him that it's a secret because then it's something that's wrong. So I won't tell him that.' She said, 'And so if he chooses then, you know, it's up to him.' So then she must deal with whatever. I don't imagine anybody will say anything, do you?
> Petra: How will that work [do you think]?
> Sally: Do you know? I don't know. (Laughs) We'll cross that bridge when we come to it. (Laughs) (411)

Sally respected her daughter's wish to keep the information hidden but did not necessarily agree that being so secretive at the start was a good strategy. Although her account is light-hearted, she remained unsure of what the consequences of having hidden this truth for so long might be for the boy when he was told. The same was true for the other families in which the donation was kept confidential. For example, Clive and Stephanie, and Danielle and Christina, planned to tell their children about the donation and Shirley knew that her grandson would eventually be told all as well. Family secrets are, of course, by no means a new phenomenon, and reproductive secrets play a prominent role in that which is kept hidden in family life (Smart, 2011). But in most circumstances, the intention is that the information will remain hidden in perpetuity. For example, a mother who falls pregnant by a man other than her husband might decide never to reveal the true paternity of the child but treat it as the child of the husband. But in the case of the families of donor conceived children, there was often an inbuilt time limit to the secret.

This meant that the future often seemed uncertain for the families in which the secrets had grown. This was highlighted with particular clarity in our interview with Sheryl, whose parents refused to tell the wider family about her ex-partner Penny, about her daughter Jennifer's conception and about the new baby sister. She found her situation very difficult and a cause of deep anxiety:

> Sheryl: I'm not having to tell anybody about stuff but I do still feel like I'm very much living this double life. (115)

It seemed clear that her secret could not be contained for much longer and yet she was not sure how to handle the situation and had not yet taken steps to tell her relatives.

> Sheryl: I don't know whether [my relatives] are kind of putting two and two together, cause they're going to in a minute because [my daughter] is going to get older and it's obviously, you know, it can't be this sort of dirty secret for ever more. I feel like I'm sitting on the fence at the moment and I don't know quite what would happen [if I told the relatives]. Yeah, I'm very much in the dark with that one because I don't know their views on things.

Although we cannot know what the future holds for these families, accounts about keeping information close reveal the difficulties that these decisions can bring about. Children, parents and grandparents, as well as other relatives, are embedded in complex family networks where lives are intimately linked together. This makes guarding and controlling the kinship information that lies at the heart of donor conception a particularly difficult task.

Conclusion

We have suggested in this chapter that sharing information about donor conception and/or lesbian parenthood can grow into an emotional and delicate issue in families, and that families can have difficulties when trying to manage and restrict the sharing of information to wider circles. To explain the complexity of the situation that emerges around such sensitivities in families, we suggest that these families juggle three distinct and yet interlinked priorities in family life.

The first priority that guides decisions to keep information restricted is the commitment to sharing information first with the child and also the perception that it is the child's personal information which he or she 'owns'. Following this line of thought, doing the right thing by the child meant protecting the information for him or her until he or she was old enough to disclose it himself or herself. Consequently, this also meant building up sensitivities in families by creating closed areas of information.

Second, parents and grandparents were concerned about the issue of privacy because they wanted to avoid social stigma. Because the conception of a child is normally a private matter parents and grandparents did not feel the need or desire to make public the specific circumstances of a donor conceived child's conception. Although lesbian couples had little possibility of hiding the fact that they have a donor conceived child, our study shows that they could nevertheless try to keep some aspects private, for example, how they conceived or who the donor was.

Third, decisions about non-disclosure were shaped by the complexity of living embedded and connected lives. This shaped the process of (non)revelation in significant ways. For example, it meant that many parents who were committed to concealment nevertheless decided to tell grandparents because they were important people in their and their child's lives. Conversely, it meant that grandparents had a stake in the decisions that were made about disclosure, and also in creating the sensitivities in the first place. Families of donor conceived children juggled these priorities, and in doing so made difficult judgement calls about how to manage their situation in the best possible way. In Chapter 5 we go on to explore what happens when families decide early on that they will be open about donor conception.

5
Opening Up: Disclosure, Information and Family Relationships

Introduction

This chapter is about the idea of openness in family relationships and explores parents' experiences of actively sharing information about donor conception with their children and with their wider family. Openness in the context of donor assisted conception has come to mean the practice whereby parents tell their children all about the means of their conception, including the role of the donor and the meaning of gamete donation. The value of providing children with this information has become an important ethical issue in the UK in recent years. The sentiment has grown that donor conceived children have the right to know about their genetic (donor) origins and that it is in their best interest to be told as much as possible about their conception as early as possible (Guichon *et al.*, 2012; Nuffield Council on Bioethics, 2013). This development has been mirrored by an academic interest in exploring how parents can be encouraged to disclose information to their children, and how society can and should act to promote disclosure (Lalos *et al.*, 2007; Blyth *et al.*, 2009; Cowden, 2012). Alongside these developments, there is an increasing body of research exploring the extent to which parents talk openly to their children about their donor origins (e.g. Daniels *et al.*, 1995, 2011; Gottlieb *et al.*, 2000; Murray and Golombok, 2003; Landau and Weissenberg, 2010; Isaksson *et al.*, 2011; Laruelle *et al.*, 2011; Appleby *et al.*, 2012).

This shift towards openness between parents and children on such intimate issues represents a radical change in the social and cultural perception of how donor conception should be managed, and this is something that is most clearly illustrated by the backdrop of secrecy that surrounded donor conception in the past. When sperm donation was first introduced in the UK as a solution to infertility in the 1930s and 1940s it was deeply controversial (Richards *et al.*, 2012). Donor insemination was never a criminal offence, although an expert advisory committee suggested in 1948 that it should be. In 1960 a UK Government Departmental Committee decided that the practice should not be prohibited but strongly discouraged (Richards *et al.*, 2012:6f.). Due to the stigma that came to be associated with sperm donation, parents of donor conceived children were encouraged to keep it secret. As assisted reproductive technologies developed in the 1970s and 1980s and reproductive donation became a more common solution to involuntary childlessness, secrecy remained the dominant pattern and parents were encouraged to not tell their children about the means of their conception (Kirkman, 2003). The recent shift away from non-disclosure towards openness was motivated in part by the parallels drawn with adoption where openness has been established practice since the 1970s (Turkmendag, 2012; see Chapter 1). With the enactment of the Human Fertilisation and Embryology Act of 2008, parents of donor conceived children were increasingly urged to adopt the new policy of disclosure.

It is important to remember, however, that this shift in the ethical guidelines for parents has come about surprisingly quickly. The idea of non-disclosure had become well embedded and the recent turnaround in advice goes against a lot of basic assumptions held by both the parent and the grandparent generation. This means not only that there may be resistance to the new values but also that there is not yet a widely accepted social narrative for translating the idea of openness into practice. Culturally speaking, there is a gap between the desire to talk openly about donor conception and the practice of doing this in families. To some extent the UK Donor Conception Network (DCN) has stepped in to fill this void.[1] Advocating openness, the DCN runs workshops about how to share information for people who are in the early stages of considering using other gametes and also for parents of existing donor conceived children. They have also developed reading material, such as children's books, to assist parents in the process of telling. However, more broadly, there are no culturally established ways for heterogeneous families in a multicultural and multi-faith society to 'do' openness and there are no common narratives to access when negotiating the process of sharing information about donor conceived children's genetic background.

In this chapter we ask what happens when families confront the duty of openness in everyday life. We explore how those who are committed to candidness negotiate what it means and what it is like to establish open lines of communication about donor conception within their families. We begin the chapter by exploring parents' views on the need for openness and we then go on to explore their experiences of sharing information with their children and how they establish frankness in relationships with relatives. In the last section we return to the parents and ask what life is like 'after openness'.

Committed to openness

The majority of parents in our study strongly believed that they needed to tell their children that they were donor conceived. We do not know, of course, how typical this is of all the parents who decide to use donor gametes but what our sample can tell us is exactly what the process is like for parents who are committed to the new ethic of openness. Victoria and her husband, for example, had two children through sperm donation and her account is indicative of how parents viewed the issue of openness, a stance which often emerged through talking to clinical staff about the issue:

> Victoria: [The counsellors at the clinic] talked about the fact that people usually tell [the children], or that the advice is to tell I think they said, and my initial reaction I think was like most people's, which is, 'Oh, it almost seems like why do you need to?' And then it's so obvious I think when you [have talked about it]. So very early on we were very clear and comfortable about the fact that absolutely the best thing was to tell. (212)

The heterosexual parents in our study typically developed a commitment to telling their children through the process of infertility counselling at clinics or they had been persuaded by the DCN. Many had been warned about the negative effects of accidental disclosure later in life and were encouraged to think of donor conception as a story about their child's origin which he or she had the right to know.

These parents thus received a powerful moral message that disclosure was in the best interest of their child; the decision about openness was often motivated by the desire to do what they perceived to be the proper thing. The lesbian parents often shared this view, but as we have already noted, they knew that they had little option but to be open and explain their families to their children.

Sharing information with children

Although parents were committed to the idea of being open it was not necessarily easy for them to translate the principle into practice. One of the reasons why they struggled with the process of telling was because they themselves had mixed feelings about having used a donor. James and Delia, for example, had a one-year-old daughter through sperm donation. James, who we discussed in some detail in Chapter 2, struggled hard to accept that he was not his daughter's genetic father. Both parents were convinced that the daughter needed to know about her donor origins, and yet James was unsure how he would be able to handle having that conversation with her:

> James: I'm going to be in that circumstance where, you know, who's going to tell [our daughter] because I feel really awkward about it still....I'm not comfortable about the fact that I'm not really her genetic father. It doesn't sit comfortably with me at all.
> Delia: And we have talked, you know, because James even a couple of weeks ago was saying, 'You're going to have to tell [her]. You're going to have to bring it up in conversation and explain why I can't talk to her about it at the moment.' (203)

It is not difficult to see that telling the story about donor conception could be highly emotionally charged if the donor conception was lodged in unresolved dilemmas about genetic relationality. It was common that the parents struggled with the process of telling because they themselves struggled to accept using a donor in the first place.

Parents also found the process challenging because they were unsure of what, how and when to tell their children. Jessica and Amy became parents of twins through IVF and donor sperm, and their children were three and a half years old at the time of the interview. They had not talked to them about the donor or the IVF and were unsure about when to do so and what to say:

> Jessica: I think it is quite important [to tell them], it's just finding the right time, the right way. I still think we will.... I guess by the time they ask questions about other children I'd like to think they've got an answer by then, I don't know. I'd hate for them to say, 'Well, two mummies can't [have children],' you know because [they get asked], 'Who's your daddy?'.... I want to be able to give them a story, an answer that isn't either untrue but also isn't about sperm and test tubes, I don't know the reason for that. (101)

Jessica wanted to tell the children a story that explains and legitimates having two mothers and no father. But at the same time she was not sure about when to tell the children and how best to do so, and she felt that the terminology such as IVF and sperm did not provide the story that she wanted to tell. Like Jessica, many others found it difficult to know when to tell the children; also, if they disclosed when the children were very young, this raised difficult issues about what words to use. Explaining donor conception meant that parents had to talk about how babies were made and it left few alternatives to explaining about sperm, eggs, sex, body parts, donors and being a lesbian. This was felt to be very challenging in relationships with young children. Lesbian couples who knew specifically that other people, as well as their own children, would bring questions to them still felt unsure about how to talk about the composition of their families. For example, Danielle knew that it was only a matter of time before the question would be asked, and yet she was not sure about how to respond:

> Danielle: I'm aware now of the fact that any time [our son] could just turn round and say, 'Do I have a daddy? Do I not have a daddy? Why not?' And at the moment I would still be a little bit stuck for an answer. (106)

This contemporary emphasis on telling created a great deal of common ground between the experiences of heterosexual and lesbian couples because they were both seeking acceptable answers to difficult questions.

In this context of uncertainty, many turned to the DCN for support. The DCN advocates that parents should tell their children when they are still very young and that they should start even when they are babies. Their children's book entitled *My Story* is a picture book which explains donor conception in child-friendly language and it is designed to be read aloud to provide a simple account of origins. Many of the heterosexual parents we interviewed mentioned having told their children about their donor origins by reading to them from the *My Story* book. Typically, parents would start reading this to their children from a very young age, often as young as six months.

> Zoe: I can remember changing [my eldest son's] nappy and saying, (long pause) the words from the *My Story* [book] . . . . You know, he was only, he could hardly sit up. Perhaps just five or six months, he was looking at the book, and I'd be in tears doing it. But then I got used to doing it and then thinking, this is silly. (202)
>
> Lea: Well I'm already telling her [two year old daughter] the story now so we'll just continue with the same [*My Story*] book . . . . I started when she was maybe six months old and you just do it for your own sake so you know how to phrase it in words. (206)

These accounts suggest that reading *My Story* aloud gave the parents a narrative with which to tell the basics to their children. It provided a script to follow and, because it was a printed book, it was a story that could be read and told in exactly the same way over and over again. But our accounts also indicate that the book provided the parents with the chance to practice how to tell the story in a context where they would otherwise struggle for words. *My Story* thus set out what to tell their children and also how to tell them; it provided a way for negotiating the telling process. Other parents created their own stories that could work in a similar fashion. Nina and Claudia had, for example, drawn a family tree on their computer that was going to be part of their baby's homemade 'life story' book.

> Nina: [The family tree] was about, really, us just being as honest as we could from the outset, which is what all the rest of this stuff

[shows on the screen] is about as well. It's just letters that we've written to the baby as we've gone along in terms of how we're feeling about the process and things. And the idea is to create a life story book. (116)

These accounts indicate how practices of telling in donor conception families borrow from more established practices in adoption, and how the creation of life story books and even memory boxes can be seen as appropriate in both situations (Sales, 2012). This is perhaps one of the clearest examples of how adoption practices have come to shape the process of openness in donor conception.

Being open with a small child about donor conception was, however, not a straightforward process. After parents had resolved to tell their children and found a way of doing so, they then had to manage the way that their children made sense of the story. Often they did so in ways which were both bewildering and surprising to their parents. Nicholas and Martha had a six-year-old son through egg donation:

Nicholas: [Our son] doesn't ask us about it particularly. But for a long time, he'd play in the mornings when he used to come into bed with us. He used to have this sort of game he played where he was hatching out of an egg. And I think in some ways, not necessarily because it was anything to do with donor conception, but because we had taken the trouble to explain to him donor conception and how he'd come about, you have to explain about eggs and sperms. And so he probably knew more about this at a much earlier age than a lot of children. And he'd invented this sort of idea around it that he hatched out of an egg because, to him, an egg is a thing with a shell around it. And he'd seen wildlife programmes about birds and lizards and any kind of animal hatched out of an egg, because all mammals start from eggs.

Martha: He does sometimes still say, 'When I hatched out of my egg'. I think it was *my* egg. I mean, maybe that's just his way of dealing with it. You know, taking that on board, that there was something unusual about his egg. (205)

Parents who went through the process of talking to their children about their family found it hard to discern what their children took from the conversation. Thus, openness threw up difficult questions about how children made sense of the information and how best to guide them in using the knowledge and the vocabulary that they were learning. Being open with a small child took parents into unknown territories as it led to situations with which they were unfamiliar. The following account from Meredith, who had two sons together with Priscilla, is illustrative of the perplexing process of explaining details about the family to a young child and guiding them in their understanding of their family structure:

> Meredith: I tried to explain what the word lesbian meant ages ago [to our five-year-old son] and I thought 'It totally hasn't gone in.' And then the other night he was getting ready for his bath and he took his vest off and put it on his head pretending it was girly hair and said, 'I'm a lesbian, I'm a lesbian girl.' And I was like, 'Do you know what a lesbian is?' and he's like, 'It's a girly, girly, girly,' and I was like, 'That could be an answer' (laughter). And I explained what one was and he was like, 'Oh . . .', and I said, 'The thing is, it's a grown-ups' word, it's probably not a good word to say at school because I bet other kids won't know what a lesbian is, they just don't understand. But you say it [to] your teacher or any grown-up you like but I don't think it's worth saying it to another kid,' and he was like, 'Oh, grown-ups' word.' And I thought, 'Oh no, it's not swearing though' (laughter). Because I don't want him to go to school going on about lesbians, it's not nice for other parents to have to deal with something they might not have to deal with is it? But at the same time I don't want him to think it's a [bad word]. So it's just like, 'Oh my god, how do you deal with it?' So he's going, 'I'm a lesbian,' (laughter) so all he picked up was a lesbian's something only a girl could be, that's all he picked up. All that explaining, all that like 'Ooooh' . . . (113)

Meredith's account indicates how difficult it can be to explain an unconventional family arrangement to a young child, and also how she tried to take account of how her son might start using the words that were being introduced. It appears she sought to balance the need to explain to her son what a lesbian was with the fact that it was not a word that young children typically know or use. She also imagined that should it enter into the children's vocabulary it would become something that could cause problems or difficulties for other parents.

And yet, the concept was, of course, fundamental to her family and so it was also an important word to get to grips with. Meredith tried to deal with this dilemma by suggesting that the little boy saw it as a grown-ups' word but that led to another difficulty. In this family, we must imagine, the children were discouraged from using swear words because they too were described as grown-ups' words. After having done much painstaking navigating and explaining to her son, she realised that all he had understood was that a lesbian was a girl. In this way, explaining about an unusual family arrangement to a small child is a challenging prospect to a parent, and it is also a process that they have to revisit time and time again as the child grows up and his or her understanding develops.

One particularly important aspect of telling a child that the parents in our study had to take into consideration was that their son or daughter might themselves start sharing the information more widely. Many parents worried about the reactions their children would receive as a consequence and so sought to construct a supportive atmosphere by sharing the information pre-emptively with their family and wider social circles.

Abigail: We've got a newish circle of friends around at the moment, you know, mums and toddlers. People with kind of similar approaches and I really value that. So somehow it came up in conversation and they know. Because he might want to say 'I came from [a donor's] egg' to them. And I don't want them to have to handle that weirdly. For them to say, 'Oh yeah, that's right, that was lucky wasn't it?' or, 'She's a kind lady'.... Making sure that the kind of environment he finds himself in is sympathetic and supportive to his musings. Even if it's just things like, you know, for a while we were reading the *My Story* book and it's all about an egg, the egg [donor] gave us an egg. And he was, for about six weeks or eight weeks, nonstop in and out of the fridge for eggs; carrying eggs around. And I'd realised that he was trying to make a connection about eggs because eggs were in the story (laughter). And you know, so even if it's just where people don't mind that he opens their fridge and says I've got an egg. (222)

It was of paramount importance to the parents that others received their children in a positive way and that they did not respond with negative judgement or disapproval. Many parents therefore found that the decision to share information with their children involuntarily propelled them into a process of sharing information more widely.

Sharing information with relatives

One particularly important audience for disclosure was the wider family. In part this was because relationships with relatives and especially parents and siblings are an important aspect of personal life (Smart, 2007) and their role is often especially significant in the context of child birth and reproduction. But, in addition, parents were keen to create a context in which their children could talk about their donor origins and feel supported and accepted.

We found, however, that telling members of the wider family about the donor conception was not necessarily an easy task. One of the reasons for this was that by sharing information about donor conception with wider family, parents also inadvertently initiated deeply intimate conversations. For some, this made the prospect of sharing information with their families truly daunting. This was illustrated in our interview with Erin, who had an egg-donor conceived child together with her husband Adam (who did not take part in the interview). Erin and Adam had decided to tell their daughter about the egg donor, and so they felt that it was necessary to tell the grandparents. But Erin conveys here how Adam struggled with the idea of telling:

> Erin: [Adam] just really struggled [with telling his family] and just didn't really want [to]. He's just not kind of good at sharing his emotions or anything; he's a very closed book and his family's not particularly close and he hadn't told them that we'd even been having fertility treatment. So I was thinking, 'Oh god it's just going to be a massive landslide of stuff, they're going to get.' 'Okay we've been struggling to have a baby, and okay we've tried IVF three times and we didn't tell you and we've done all this stuff and we never kind of invited you in and now we're just going to hit you with this, like. By the way, Erin's pregnant and it's donor conceived.' I just thought that's a lot for them to kind of take on board. But I just thought you've got to do

it, we've got to do it, there's no choice, we've got to do it, get on with it. And eventually he did, he wrote to his parents. Just couldn't bring himself to sort of talk to them about it, so he kind of came up with the only path that he thought he could manage.... Yeah [so] he wrote to his parents and I can't remember, did they write back? Oh god I think, you know what I think, they texted, (laughs). I think they sent him a text...to say we have received your letter and...What did they say?...I think they wanted to say 'Yes we have got your letter and we have read it and we understand'....And you won't be surprised to hear that we haven't talked about it with them since. (217)

Adam was the child's genetic father and so his concern with sharing information was not about conveying to his parents that their grandchild-to-be was genetically unrelated to them. His reluctance to tell his parents did not seem to be linked to a fear of rejection or disapproval either. What appears to have been so challenging for Adam was the process of revealing intimate information. The process raised difficulties because it meant taking family relationships into unknown territories. Adam's concerns about telling would seem to indicate that this family handled intimate issues through tactful silences and avoidance. So where silence has become the established way of managing intimacy over many years, to suddenly instigate a very intimate conversation in the way that Adam felt that he had to do, was experienced as deeply uncomfortable. The account brings to mind Finch and Mason's (1993) finding that non-discussion and not explicitly talking about things in families is an important strategy through which they manage potentially difficult or contentious issues (see also Ponse, 1976). It seems Adam felt unable or unwilling to talk to his family about the issue for many years, thus highlighting how a lack of openness played a powerful role in his family network. The account also shows how openness could feel so fraught that the topic was never again revisited. Many of the parents we spoke to shared Adam's experience and so struggled with undertaking the process of telling itself.

Creating open lines of communication about donor conception in families could also be difficult because kin were fundamentally opposed to the very method of conception (Lorbach, 2003). This was illustrated in our interview with Julia and Molly, who had discussed the conception of their children with Molly's family and had received unsupportive responses from both her father and sister. Julia recalls the conversation with Molly's sister in which this emerged:

> Julia: I remember having a conversation with [your sister] about your dad's feelings about [our son] and the nature of his conception and [your sister] said something like, 'But it's just something that we just don't want to talk about.' As if [our son] being produced by donor insemination was...something rather unpleasant, and, you know, 'We'd rather not talk about that because it's not very nice'....It was almost like, this is something that shouldn't really have happened or it's a problem that needs to be fixed or a problem that we can't fix so we just brush it under the carpet and we don't discuss it.
>
> Molly: But I think we have to [keep silent], that's the situation and we know that that exists so we do brush it under the carpet because I think we're all old enough and lovely enough to know that if we ever did bring it up that would be another relationship that would be scuppered. So I would rather keep that 10 per cent of it away in order to have the 90 per cent of the whole family knowing each other and [our children]; having the cousins and that support. (103)

Molly and Julia felt that in order to preserve vital relationships with family members they had little choice but to avoid the topic of donor conception. Openness about controversial topics can cut at the heart of family life and this account is suggestive of the difficult compromises that some couples felt they had to make, such as not mentioning the donor conception in order to maintain good relationships with family. A tacit agreement not to discuss the donor conception enabled family relationships to continue despite the underlying disagreement.

Parents also struggled to create an open atmosphere about the donor conception because although they wanted to discuss the issue frankly, the older generation might fail to understand why discussing it was so important. This was illustrated in our interview with Holly and Patrick, who were convinced that candid conversations about the donor conception was extremely important for their son, but found that the paternal grandparents did not see the issue in the same light:

> Holly: When he was young, we kept having those conversations [with Patrick's parents]. 'How do you now feel about it? Have you had any thoughts about the process?' And they didn't appear to have had any thoughts about it really. No, well, I think eventually [Patrick's] dad, ... said, 'He's here, he's great. What's the problem?' Effectively, 'What are you going on about it for?' ... 'Because we have a duty to. Because we need to go on with him being open about his origins and as his knowledge and understanding becomes greater we have to respond in an appropriate way, so we have to keep learning and keeping up with his development and whatever. It isn't over and done with. We have a child; we all love him to bits but there's an extra dimension to our family .... So, we need you on board, singing from the same hymn sheet. We need you to give the same message that we have learned.' (218)

Although parents took on board the modern message of openness, wider family could perceive the issue, and how it should be managed, quite differently. In this family, the grandparents did not share the parents' sentiment and appeared to have a different approach to what was important in family life and how family relationships should be managed. Many of the grandparents we spoke to were delighted to become grandparents, but found their son's and daughter's views on openness and ongoing discussion about the donor origins unnecessary or even a pointless burden for a small child. Holly's account about struggling with her parents-in-law can be understood as a battle over meaning in a situation where there was no intergenerational agreement on the best thing to do. In this context we can understand Holly's frustration with getting her parents-in-law to 'sing from the same hymn sheet' while also understanding the older generation's dismay.

An additional reason why parents struggled to establish openness with relatives was that although they themselves accepted their inability to conceive a child together and felt relaxed talking about it, family members were less comfortable. It was common for parents to find that a relative who had been told, in subsequent meetings did not appear to have understood the significance of donor conception, or to remember having been told. Elizabeth and Adrian had a son of 18 months through sperm donation because Adrian was infertile. They spoke openly about Adrian's condition and the genetic background of their son but found it hard to communicate this issue to the boy's genetic grandmother, as she seemed quite unwilling to take on board the personal information about Adrian.

> Elizabeth: Oh, my mum doesn't deal with it very well at all. [M]y mum... keeps saying, 'Oh, perhaps he's Adrian's anyway.'
> Adrian: And, 'You don't have to tell him, you can just bring him up and just pretend that it's....'... And it's having to constantly tell her that that's not what we're doing. [Our son is] being told, even from now... so he grows up much more relaxed.
> Petra: Right, so have you sort of had a few clashes with her around it? (Both Adrian and Elizabeth laugh)
> Elizabeth: Oh, she's terrible. No, I think nowadays, the clashes tend to be: she'll say something and then one of us will very firmly put her back in her place and say, 'No, that's not how it is.' So yes, there's been various conversations of, 'No, he is going to know,' or, 'No, it's definitely that,' or she goes, 'Oh, perhaps he is Adrian's,' and we're like, 'No, he's a donor baby because Adrian can't father children that way.' (221)

A combination of processes appears to be at work in this family. We cannot know how the grandmother herself perceived the situation, but interestingly, the ongoing controversy did not appear to be about the use of sperm donation as such, but rather about how the donation should be managed and understood in the family subsequently. The grandmother appears to be of the view that donor conception is better forgotten about, and by hanging on to what she perceives to be a slight possibility that Adrian did in fact father the child, she can more easily discount the donor conception and the need to discuss it at all. Elizabeth's mother was also one of the grandparents who were unwilling to tell the rest of the family about the donor conception (see Chapter 4). Perhaps by trying to negotiate with Elizabeth and Adrian about the truth of the genetic background of the child, she was hopeful that the issue need never be discussed and that rest of the family did not need to find out. From Adrian and Elizabeth's point of view, however, the grandmother's unwillingness to adopt the same story about donor conception as they did caused frustration and also blocked their attempts to establish openness on the issue in the wider family. In families where grandparents or other relatives appeared unable to understand or even remember the donation, and where the parents did not insist on pushing the conversation, it might never be known whether the issue was really grasped. In cases where euphemisms such as 'fertility baby' were routinely used, it might mean a family member did not understand the details about the donation, or that he or she was coping with the situation by simply ignoring the whole thing.

After openness

In the last section of this chapter we turn our attention to the parents themselves and ask what it was like for them to live with the disclosure once openness had been established. One illustration comes from our interview with Vanessa, a lesbian mother of three. She had conceived twins with the help of a known sperm donor, Martin. Martin was the partner of one of her brothers, Edward, and so Martin was at the same time the children's uncle-in-law and their genetic donor/father. She had conceived the children at a time when she was in a same-sex relationship but this had subsequently broken down when the children were still very young. This meant that Vanessa became a single mother and so her parents and siblings became more involved. Vanessa's other brother Andrew, for example, took an active role in supporting her and her children. However, an incident caused a rift in their relationships and resulted in Vanessa seeking a greater distance from him:

Vanessa: Andrew was much more involved in the beginning but then, you know, the last time he was ever invited to any of the children's birthday parties, where there were actually children present, was their fifth birthday party and he sat down next to a parent at school who I had barely exchanged five words with and informed her, pointing to Martin, that he was their biological father. So I then had to have a conversation with a woman whose name I didn't even know at school about the fact that, yes, he was their biological father but the children didn't yet know the fact and I would like her to treat it as confidential for the next five years. He just doesn't have any sense, so he's a bit of a wild card.... (104)

Parents being open did not mean that they were happy for information about donor conception to be shared indiscriminately. Instead, they were often careful about who they told and also about how others, in turn, handled their information. They balanced openness with wanting (and needing) to maintain private boundaries. Vanessa's account about Andrew sharing information too widely indicates that the meaning of donor conception, and how it should be managed, is carefully and cautiously negotiated in families and a breach of the appropriate boundaries can have severe consequences for family relationships.

Ultimately, however, once information was shared with their children or with their family members, parents were unable to control the process any longer (Lorbach, 2003). Through our interviews with parents who had started to have dialogues about donor conception, it became apparent that from that moment onwards, they were unable to steer the process of openness. Life after openness thus meant, from the parents' point of view, that they were not in control of information that was deeply personal and private. They were unable to be selective about keeping this aspect of their private lives hidden from public view (or scrutiny). Vanessa went on to reflect on Andrew's behaviour and the drawbacks of openness:

> Vanessa: I wouldn't trust him as far as I could throw him in terms of [telling people], I'm sure he's told tons of friends of his all sorts of stuff I would rather they didn't know but you know once the, arghh, once the ball starts rolling you can't control it anymore. People like to imagine that they can control all these things but you can't. Because there's always someone you tell and what they do with it is their thing and that's kind of the disadvantage of being as open as I am.

Life after openness meant that parents were unable to maintain their own private boundaries and to be selective about how sensitive information concerning their family life was dispersed publicly.

For many parents, frankness brought with it difficult decisions about how to balance openness with their own and their children's need for privacy.

Conclusion

In this chapter we have explored how parents deal with the task of being open in everyday life and how they negotiate that process in the absence of established or accepted cultural narratives about donor conception. Our exploration of how parents negotiate openness, what they say and how their message is received by their children and families sheds light on the complexities embedded in this process, showing that the practical implementation of the idea of openness is not an easy task. To conclude, we want to highlight three particular aspects of our findings.

First, we suggest that openness, in the context of donor conception, needs situating in the practicalities of everyday life. We argue that rather than seeing disclosure as a one-off occasion in which information is passed on from one person to another, it is more relevant to talk about openness as a process of establishing open lines of communication but that these lines are shaped by existing family relationships. Many parents found it immensely difficult to create a situation in their families in which the donor conception could be explicitly discussed. Sharing information with their children was a challenging task, not least because it was a process that had to be revisited as the child's knowledge and understanding developed. Sharing information with family members could also be immensely difficult and there was no agreed method to fall back on as a way of managing the process. Importantly, we found that families might share information about donor conception but without having the chance to establish a common or shared system of values first. For example, sharing information about donor conception in a family with an established culture of not sharing private or intimate details could mean taking a step into the unknown. In other families, where relatives disapproved, silence on the matter appeared the only way of maintaining family relationships. Thus addressing the elephant in the room could cause problems and make relationships very awkward. For this reason in particular, in many families donor conception became a topic that, once mentioned, was never raised again. We therefore suggest that information sharing needs to be understood as a relational process which unfolds along the lines of already established ways of relating and in accordance with existing family biographies. There is, we discovered, an important difference between information being transmitted and communication being established. To understand openness in the context of donor conception, we must therefore situate it in people's actual lives and family relationships.

Second, this chapter highlights how the move towards disclosure in the field of donor conception challenges boundaries between people's private and public lives. Both heterosexual and lesbian donor conception propel these private matters into a more public sphere. Deeply personal facts about genetic linkages or disconnections, donation, sexuality, infertility and (non-viable) sperm or eggs enter into the public realm. This makes parents' intimate and personal life more exposed, and more vulnerable, to public scrutiny. With disclosure, the parents sacrifice aspects of their private life and forgo the power to draw their own and their family's boundaries of acceptable privacy. The consequences of such openness could be very difficult to negotiate as parents lost control over their own information and how it was shared.

Lastly, the stories we heard about disclosure might have been specifically about donor conception, but they also shed light on wider aspects of family relationships. Donor conception, like a prism, brings into relief varied and multilayered aspects of family relationships. Family life was revealed as a potentially risky business. In everyday families people do not always communicate openly or even love each other deeply. They may disapprove of each other or simply be fairly indifferent. Children may not feel a debt of duty to parents and not all parents may feel they must be endlessly supportive of their children. It is in this context of the actual families we live with that donor conception parents must manage their own and their children's identities. Lesbian mothers could not automatically assume that their parents would be delighted to learn of the birth of a donor conceived grandchild and heterosexual parents could not take for granted that grandparents would accept a non-genetic grandchild. Our interviews with parents who struggled to instigate deeply personal conversations with their own parents suggest that closeness can be absent just when it is most needed. Although many couples found support from someone inside their wider family, they quickly found out who they could trust or who they wanted to trust with intimate details of their lives. It is this complex pattern of relationships which we argue must always be taken into account when understanding how people deal with the new phenomenon of donor conception.

6
Relating to Donors: Strangers, Boundaries and Tantalising Knowledge

Introduction

In this chapter we discuss the complex ways in which families of donor conceived children make sense of the child's genetic connection outside the family to the egg, sperm or embryo donor(s). The donor relationship raises difficult questions, for example, how the donor should relate to the family and the child, his or her role in child's life and also how the child relates to other donor kin connections, for example donor siblings. In this chapter we explore how families perceive and negotiate the donor relationship and donor connections as part of their everyday family life.

The parents in our study conceived using both unknown and known donors. It was most common that couples conceived using an unknown donor and 70 per cent (or 31 out of 44) of our parents had conceived using such a donor.[1] This was linked to the fact that the majority of the couples we interviewed had accessed donor gametes through licensed clinics. In the introduction we discussed in detail how donation is organised in clinics in the UK, but here it is sufficient to note that reproductive health care centres in the UK are set up so that donors are unknown to the recipients. This means that no social relationship travels along the lines of the genetic contribution made by the donor and, at the time of donation, contact between the donor, the donor's family and the receiving parents is unachievable. As we noted in the introduction, in the UK children conceived after 1 April 2005 have the right to seek out the identity of the donor when they reach 18, but before that age the donor's identity remains unknown to them as well. These somewhat enigmatic relationships stand in stark contrast to known donor relationships where people arrange the donation themselves. Thirty per cent, or 13 couples, in our study had conceived using a known donor. In such arrangements, the parties know each other personally; they have met at least once or can be good friends or even family. Often the donation in such cases is a personal gift from the donor to the intended parents. Rather than this being a remote, even unknowable relationship, these parents and donors know one another and many have a level of involvement in one another's lives.

It might be assumed that for couples who conceive using an unknown donor, he or she would cease to be particularly meaningful after conception precisely because no relationship can be forged. However, we found that parents (and grandparents) do form an imaginary or, as we shall now call it, an enigmatic relationship with their donor as their children grew up. We found that this enigmatic relationship introduced curious questions in the minds of parents and novel situations in their lives, which meant that the donor continued to have a presence after the birth. Parents who conceived in known donor situations also continued to relate to their donors, but we found that the ongoing issues raised in these families were quite different and so we discuss them separately. We begin by exploring relationships with the enigmatic donor and address issues such as how he or she can acquire an 'absent presence' in the life of the family, how parents deal with the possibility of unknown donor siblings and how they manage potential kinship connections as part of their everyday lives. We also address how knowing about the enigmatic donor is both tantalising and yet unthinkable. In the second half of the chapter we address known donor relations. We explore this relationship as a conduit for relatedness with the donor and his or her own family and also how parents negotiate boundaries between their and the donor's families. Finally we investigate how personal relationships develop over time in the context of known donations and how that can shape and change relationships.

Relating to unknown donors

An absent presence

Cathryn: There was a phase..., the first year I think of [both of my girls'] babyhood where the donor was a bit like a ghost in the

room. And there was like another person around, but they don't
have a face or a shape. And you're looking, a bit like everybody
does, looking at babies and go... 'Who are they like?' And with
[our eldest], I remember going through a phase where I'd think,
because I didn't know anything about being a parent or what to
do or about little kids anyway, she'd do something or behave in
a certain way and I'd think... 'Where's this come from?' almost.
And I think if she was mine genetically I'd still think 'Where has
this come from?' (laughs). (201)

Cathryn and Daniel had two daughters by egg donation and the girls
had been conceived using two different unknown donors. As Cathryn
embarked on motherhood, she remarked that she could feel the presence of the egg donors in the room. By using the metaphor of a
ghost she conjured up an image of two spectres that she could not
see or know, although she felt their presence very powerfully. Grace
et al. (2008) found similar accounts, in their interviews, of unknown
donors where the donor remained a 'shadowy figure' in the life of
the family, a figure who never materialised because so little could be
known about them. To Cathryn, the presence of the donor emerged
as she was asking herself questions about who her babies were like.
Genes and blood are perceived culturally as prominent markers of
personhood and belonging, and this belief translates into numer-
ous practices, including mapping and explaining a person's looks and
character through his or her genetic relationships (Becker *et al.*, 2005;
Mason, 2008; Marre and Bestard, 2009; Nordqvist, 2010). The presence of the donor in Cathryn's mind was thus motivated by broader
cultural ideas linking personhood and genetic inheritance, leading
her to see and make connections between the children and the donor.

This account is illustrative of one of the ways that an unknown
egg or sperm donor acquired an enigmatic presence in some families, namely through the developing character of the children. Many
parents and grandparents shared these kinds of questions about what
the donor was like. Cara, for example, wondered whether her daughter's strong abilities in maths had come from the donor, and many
grandparents admitted to feeling very curious about who the donor
was and what he or she was like.

The donor could also acquire this enigmatic presence in the minds
of families with children from donor identity release programmes

because he or she was seen as a character waiting in the wings as the child grew up, potentially ready to emerge as the child reached 18. This potential reappearance of the donor could have consequences for the parents who felt unable to leave the issue of the donation behind. James, for example, struggled with being a non-genetic father through sperm donation, and ultimately found the idea of his daughter seeking out the donor very difficult to cope with:

> James: I guess her donor then can be identified when she's 18.... Don't want anything to do with it, is how I feel right now. But we're not there, so anything can change. And that's how I cope with it. I hope that she doesn't feel the need [to seek him out].... You know, we will have had 18 years of daddy and daughter, and all of a sudden Genetic Man pops up on the scene. I don't know. I mean, you know, I've always had this feeling that if I met him I'd want to kill him. (203)

For James and several others, the donation raised unresolved feelings and these were kept alive in part because of the possibility of later identity release. It appears that James felt very threatened by the donor while others felt ambivalence and uncertainty and, in this way, the donor continued to be the focus of unhelpful thoughts and anxieties.

The absent presence of the donor thus lingered on in a perpetually unsatisfactory way which meant that the donation gave rise to feelings among parents that they could never resolve. As Monica Konrad argues, this unfinished experience can be understood as an outcome of the process of concealment. The unknown donor is a relationship which is characterised by actively keeping the identities of the donor and the recipients hidden from one another. Konrad (2005:180) suggests that this active form of 'not knowing' creates an unfinished relationship simply because so little is known about the other party. Paradoxically, thinking about the unknown donor produces the ongoing presence of the donor in the life of the donor conceived family.

Donor siblings

Many parents of children conceived using unknown donor gametes wrestled with another unfinished aspect of the donation, which was the idea of potential donor siblings. By virtue of the donor connection, the donor conceived child could have a number of unknown half-siblings growing up in other families. Many parents found the idea of their existence and any potential future relationship between their own children and these siblings disquieting. Molly and Julia, for example, had two children as a result of licensed identity release donor sperm. In general they felt comfortable about the way they had been conceived but the thought of siblings continued to disturb them:

> Molly: There's one element of it all that still slightly freaks me out, which is that there are other children. And that is a big, it doesn't slightly freak me out, there's something that I kind of suppress all the time, that there are half-siblings. That's the whole bit that I find very...
> Julia: Murky?
> Molly: ...yeah, it's just, there's something that I feel instinctively is wrong with that.... I find really, it's something just odd about it. Just really, that, 'Do you see what I mean?' That whole element is so...dark. There's something really, I can't find the word, I don't know what the word is, but there's something quite disturbing about it. That whole kind of unresolved, that's one aspect that will always be unresolved... (103)

Molly and Julia half knew that it was likely that there would be other children out there to whom their own children were genetically related. The issue of donor siblings was, in the words of Konrad (2005:180), therefore a known 'half known'. Kevin, who had two children from donated sperm together with Erica, expressed similar concerns:

> Kevin: The idea that they'll have brothers and sisters who aren't part of our family, I have a gut reaction – it's not logical. I feel (long pause), I'd rather not think about that. I'd rather that didn't happen. (209)

Currently in the UK, licensed donor gametes can be used to create ten different families (HFEA, 2013c). Within these families there is, however, no limit to the number of children that can be generated by one donor's sperm. Thus it is not inconceivable that there could be around 20 donor siblings for every donor conceived child. Cara had a teenage daughter conceived using donor sperm and she recounts her daughter's strong concern for how may donor siblings she could potentially have:

> Cara: I don't think she likes the idea of being sort of diluted. Do you know what I mean? Almost a sense of... That she's one of a production line. (Laughs). You know, it's like sort of a limited edition print. You know, how many is it? Are you one of 500? Are you one of 5000 or are you one of 15?... I don't know. Maybe it's just something like that. You know, just sort of churning out children. (220)

These sentiments imply that the possible existence of a large number of donor siblings does not fit comfortably within kinship principles where notions of individuality and uniqueness are tied in with a person's genetic inheritance. It appears that the thought of too many children born from the same donor dilutes the particularity of intergenerational genetic links and therefore individual specialness.

The idea of donor siblings, and the feeling of discomfort they inspire in both parents and donor conceived offspring, reflect an overarching dimension that characterises the donor relationship. This is that the donation of a single egg or sperm creates a genetic connection not only between the child and the donor, but also between that child and anyone else who is genetically linked to the donor. The donor conceived child's genetic connection to the donor can shift and change into something that looks quite different in form (for example a connection to donor siblings) and so the donor relationship has the ability to give rise to a vast number of potential relational possibilities. Building on this insight, Konrad (2005:49, 173) suggests that the donor relationship is a 'transilient' relationship, meaning a relationship that has the potential to leap from being one thing to becoming another. The leap from being connected to the donor to being connected to donor siblings is one example of this transilience. But it does not, of course, stop at donor siblings. The donor relationship can also become the connection between the donor conceived child and other donor kin connections, for example donor grandparents or donor aunts and uncles.

Managing enigmatic donor kinship connections

So far we have shown that the enigmatic donor relationship introduces both perpetually unresolved issues in families that travel with
them into the future and a transilient relationship that can leap from
being one thing to being another. In our interviews we found that
these aspects of the donor relationship were not only something that
occupied parents' imaginings, but could pop up unexpectedly as a
potential reality in a perfectly normal situation. Our interview with
Julia and Molly exemplifies this:

> Julia: When I was pregnant with [our son] I remember doing a
> pregnancy yoga, and there was this woman who did pregnancy
> yoga and we got chatting and it turned out that she also was a
> lesbian and she had also had used assisted reproduction through
> the same clinic and her baby was due a few months before [our
> son], and I remember suddenly having this moment where I just
> thought, 'Oh my God, she might, she might have used the same
> donor.' And I was like looking at my bump and looking at her
> bump and thinking, 'These guys might be half-siblings,' and
> I never actually, I didn't have the guts to say to her, 'So who's
> your donor?' Because I didn't wanna know, I didn't want her to
> say, 'Oh yeah, it's this guy, he's this, he's this, he's this' and I'd
> go, 'Oh my God, that's our guy. Oh my God, you know, our kids
> are actually related.' (103)

Several of our interviewees had at some point found themselves in a
situation where it was possible to seek information about the donor
or potentially to identify 'donor siblings'. Parents came in touch with
potential donor connections through everyday life activities, and this
meant that they found themselves in situations where they had to
decide whether to make these enigmatic donor connections more
tangible. Julia's decision not to ask questions that would identify
donor kinship was echoed in other parents' accounts about how they
managed such situations. We found that parents approached the possibility of new connections arising from the donation with caution;
they handled any such potential connectedness with extreme care.
Typically, they avoided making the unknown known. As illustrated in
Julia's account, parents would *actively* refrain from speaking of certain
topics or pursuing a particular relationship in order to maintain their

lack of knowledge about any potential donor relation. Thus, they were actively engaged in *not* finding out information about donors or potential siblings that were possibly within their reach. It seemed the donation threatened to lead to 'too much relationality' (Konrad, 2005:187) and a proliferation of donor kinship connections was not welcome. The parents were engaged in processes of *limiting* kinship, and they did this by leaving things unsaid or neglected. As Konrad would argue, they used delimitation as a strategy to contain the perceived excess that knowing might bring.

This is an issue that needs some consideration, given that parents of donor conceived children now organise themselves in communities such as the Donor Conception Network (DCN) and Lesbian Mums groups. Indeed Gemma, a member of the DCN, noted that this was something that members of the DCN were already managing, tacitly, within the organisation:

> There's an unknown (sic) rule at donor [conception] network that you don't talk about your donor's profiles because you could inadvertently make somebody realise your children are siblings. (114)

It is now more likely that parents will find themselves in situations where they have to make decisions about limiting, or expanding, their donor kin connections.

How might we understand the desire to limit kinship connections and the sense of danger that was perceived to lie in making the concealed donor link known? The disclosure of a genetic link between two children in different families would instantly make the children related and position them, as well as their parents and families, in a relationship with one another. A known genetic connection is irreversible (Strathern, 1995) and so the connection between genetic relatives (for example two children) could never again be unknown. Knowledge about a genetic relationships also brings with it responsibilities. Jeanette Edwards (2000:224) suggests that to be connected yet not to claim that connectedness is problematic. Thus, parents who find out about a genetic link with another family also possibly have a form of responsibility towards them. Being connected brings with it duties of contact and communication. Thus the revelation of donor kinship connections ties together families who are then left with the difficult decision of deciding what to do with that knowledge. It is not a relationship that maps onto conventional kinship and so there are no prescribed codes of conduct or etiquette. It is perhaps not surprising that parents usually decided that maintaining ignorance was the best and safest course of action.

Tantalising knowledge

While we found that conjuring up the enigmatic donor could invite unsettling thoughts and that parents would stop themselves from making kin connections known, we also found that, at the same time, knowing more about a donor was a particularly tantalising prospect. Julia told us a story about having found herself in a situation where the identity of her unknown donor had seemed within reach, and this exemplifies how exciting knowledge about the donor could seem. She decided to buy vials of frozen sperm provided by their donor from the sperm bank to be stored in case they decided to have another child. She believed that the clinic kept vials of sperm for ten years, and so on finding out that the vials she had bought actually expired after five, she called the clinic:

> Julia: I rang the clinic and spoke to this woman in the donor bank and said, 'What's going on with this, I kind of assumed that they'd all have ten years on them, and why do they only have five years on them and, you know, what's going on?' And she explained that the donor, when they donate, can make a decision about how long the expiry is, and that our donor had ticked the five year box when he'd donated. But she said to me, 'You know, that was, that was quite a while ago, and he might be willing to kind of extend it for you,' and then she said, 'Oh, I can just give him a call if you like.' And I had this sudden moment where I was like, 'Oh my God, she's got his name and his phone number on her computer screen right in front of her and she can just pick up the phone and speak to him,' and it really threw me and it was very odd just to think, 'He's out there, he's a real guy … He's out there and she can just pick up the phone and she knows his name' . . . . I got very emotional. (103)

We must imagine that in Julia's mind, the donor had been a distant, almost imaginary figure that would only become less unreal if her children decided to find out his identity after turning 18. But the phone call to the clinic brought the donor much closer, and to Julia, this was utterly strange as well as hugely fascinating. The donor's identity, which before had been screened from her, was suddenly almost within her reach, and the prospect of knowing more about him was tantalising.

Part of the reason why Julia found the exchange both shocking and enthralling was that the donor suddenly appeared to her as real. Her surprise at this revelation may at first appear strange, given that she of course knew about the donor's existence. However, her reaction can perhaps be explained by the processes that couples enter into, and become part of, within the clinic context. When entering into the clinic space, intended parents also enter into a process where the relationship with the donor is managed through an apparatus of protocols, practices and regulations. An intended consequence of this apparatus is that the parents are separated from the donors. A result of this is that the donor becomes depersonalised and less 'real' in the minds of the couple. Couples who access the clinic enter into a system which in and of itself renders the donor into a non-person (Thompson, 2001; Grace *et al.*, 2007; Nordqvist, 2011b). What the phone call did was effectively render the donor into a person for Julia.

Another example of how the donor can become real and how knowledge about him or her can be hugely tantalising emerged in our interview with Martha and Nicholas. They had a son conceived using anonymous egg donation, and they thought that they had seen the donor in the waiting room at the clinic the day of their fresh egg transfer. Although we cannot know if this was the case, their account of this meeting is illustrative of the strong feelings of excitement felt:

> Nicholas: The thing that I think probably sticks in our mind more than anything was...I think it was when you went back in after they put the eggs in. We saw a woman on the other side of the waiting room. And I think you just caught her eye....And there was a sort of, 'Click it's you' [you're the donor].
>
> Martha: We don't know for sure because you're not supposed to meet, you see. But, of course, you've both got to be there [for fresh egg donation] on the same day....
>
> Nicholas: You're both in the same clinic....In fact, they've only really got the one waiting room. So the chances are you're going

to be in the same room at the same time. And even though you don't know each other, that little paragraph [you are given about the donor], of all the people in the room, ... you think, 'Oh, that's the kind of picture I have in my mind of what the donor might look like.' And if she fits that description as far as the paragraph goes, there's a fairly high chance that that's who it was.

Martha: ... We were heading for the water cooler because you have to drink lots of water before [treatment]. She sort of looked at me and I looked at her and I thought, 'We probably didn't ought to do this,' (laughter) and we sort of smiled gently and trotted off. It may not have been her. But it might have been. She looked very nice.... So, in a way, I don't feel she's that anonymous because I have that picture of her in my mind, which is nice. (205)

As the boundary between knowing and not knowing came into question, there was a great sense of excitement and anticipation. Regardless of whether Martha and Nicholas really did see their donor, or only imagined that the woman by the water cooler was her, what emerges here is that they experienced this moment as utterly charged, emotional and enthralling. Years later, it was still a very strong and meaningful memory to them. What is also significant is that although Martha and Nicholas felt that they did have the chance to talk to her, and make themselves known, they did not take it. To do so would have meant breaking the taboo around not knowing that fundamentally shapes the enigmatic donor relationship. Nevertheless, it was a tantalising meeting which in their minds moved the donor from being unknown to being *someone*.

Relating to known donors

An open relationship with a known donor avoids the kinds of negotiations produced in the framework of not knowing described above. It introduces a completely different set of parameters because parents and donor know each other. They therefore have to negotiate the shape and form of the unusual arrangement they have together, and what that relationship means.

Of the 13 couples who had known donors, ten were lesbian couples using sperm donation and three were heterosexual couples using egg donation. In the case of sperm donation it was usually organised informally and without medical intervention. Egg donation, however, required medical assistance and could be done only within the clinic context. It is worth noting that these relationships could look very different. Known donor relations could be couples and donors who had got in touch for the purpose of donation and who had met but who were otherwise more or less strangers. But there could also be arrangements between longstanding friends or within the wider family. None of the couples in our study had entered into a co-parenting relationship with the donor or shared parenthood equally with him or her.

Known donors and conduits of relatedness

The central issue that emerged from parents' stories about having a known donor was the potential for social relationships to develop with both the donor and his or her other family members. In other words, the donor might bring with him or her connection with other children or additional grandparents, aunts and uncles. Thus the donation has the potential to open up conduits of relatedness between the couple's family and the family of the donor. There is as yet no established custom and practice to help families understand these new forms of relating or for knowing what to expect from these novel forms of kinship. This lack of clarity was illustrated in Hannah's account. She was the grandmother of an egg-donor conceived child. Her youngest daughter had been unable to conceive and, when she needed donor eggs, a cousin had offered hers. This cousin was Hannah's niece, the daughter of Hannah's brother. This meant that Hannah was at the same time the child's social grandmother and her genetic great-aunt, and her brother was at the same time the child's genetic grandfather and social great-uncle. Hannah recounted a conversation with her brother about the arrangement:

> Hannah: [My brother] turned round and said, 'Oh, what do you feel about it, Hannah?' I said, 'Well look it's not what I dreamt of but I think it's a wonderful gift [your daughter] has given us.' And I said, 'I'm really quite at ease with it.' And he said, 'Well, it'll be my grandchild, really, won't it?' I said, 'No.' I said, 'Not really. You know, it might be biologically but,' I said, 'we'll be doing all the hard work and everything else.' (401)

The connections that stemmed from known donation crossed social and genetic kinship categories, and this meant that no obvious script existed for how parents and relatives should make sense of their connections. Instead it could mean different things to different family members. Hannah and her brother both drew on cultural understandings of kinship, and yet came to very different conclusions about their own relationships to the child. Relationships that emerged in the context of known donation were therefore deeply ambiguous and it was unclear how they should be defined.

Parents and grandparents often found it difficult to cope with this lack of clarity. Misunderstandings and divergent definitions of reality could feel very disturbing for those who were anxious about the unknown potential of donor kinship connections and who wanted relationships to be understood in a particular way. Hannah (above) felt deeply troubled by the conversation with her brother and sought advice about how to manage the situation. Claims of kinship were at stake, and some families found it important to manage these negotiations so that all parties understood what were to be the correct requisites of relatedness. This was illustrated in our interview with Holly and Patrick, who had a five-year-old son. The egg donor, Gina, was a friend of Holly's, and had children of her own. Holly and Patrick were content with their relationship with Gina, but there had been 'one little blip' along the way. Holly had gleaned from Gina that, when Gina talked to her own son about having donated an egg, she had referred to Holly's son as his brother:

> Holly: I was a bit concerned that she had told her son that these two children were brothers. And I said [to her], 'Oh, I hadn't quite seen it like that really'... We talked it through and she'd obviously thought it through afterwards and said, 'Yes, you're right, they're not.' Because her youngest child has a different father, she divorced with her first husband and she said to me, 'Our child is as much a brother to [my eldest children] as their youngest brother.... My son and her youngest have her genes; they have that in common, don't they?' And I said, 'Well,... there's social relationships too, you know. Do you then feel that you're [my son's] mother?' 'Oh, no, I don't at all.' I said, 'Well, then, it's kind of the same thing. You know, that if you're not his mother then how would your child be his brother? Because it's not just about the genes, but the social, and being brought up in

the same family and things.' And she said, 'You're right, I agree. I hadn't thought it through, I hadn't thought it through'. [...] And I said 'I think we should shape for them what this relationship is. At the moment I feel it's a special connection.' And she thought about it and she said, 'You're right, it is. I feel that with him. He's not my child and I'm very clear about that but I feel a special connection with him.' I said, 'Well, it's the same for your children then. There's a special connection' .... That's what she decided she would say next time [the children asked], 'There's a special connection.' Yes, which kind of feels okay. (218)

To Holly it was very important that the connection between her son, the donor and the donor's family was not conceptualised exactly as kinship. Gina's understandable reference to the children as brothers was therefore difficult for Holly to accept. To resolve it, Holly negotiated with Gina about how to understand the connection between the children and the meaning and significance of genetic kinship and social relationships. She rejected the counter-argument that Gina's son had other half-siblings and that, genetically speaking, Holly's son was simply another half-sibling because this seemed to threaten her own status as the boy's only mother. Ultimately she suggested that the relationship should be understood as a special connection and in so doing denied the possibility that it could be defined as a form of kinship. This example shows how claims to connectedness in known donor relations can be quite problematic and also how the meaning of being connected must be carefully negotiated. We can understand both Holly's and Hannah's accounts as attempts to choreograph kinship by foregrounding the social aspects of kinship discourse and minimising the genetic ones (Thompson, 2005).

It was not always easy for parents and grandparents to manage the prospective proliferation of relatedness that could come with known donor relations. To limit excess kinship, some engaged in a process of guarding boundaries around their families. Holly further provided a good example of the need for geographical distance to help in the management of clear relationships:

Holly: Well, she's ... distant; she's about 60 miles away. If she lived round the corner we'd have to [do] much more work on that one. The clinic would have been asking us about that. I think they were quite pleased that there was this physical distance.

It would make the social, the socialising easier. We wouldn't have the children all at the same school saying, 'Oh, we're brothers,' and having to explain it all. So, I think it made things easier. (218)

The spatial distance between the families offered Holly some peace of mind and made it easier for her to interrupt the excess of relatedness the donor relationship gave rise to. There was too much at stake in allowing a social relationship based on genetic connections to grow between the children. In her mind the lack of a social relationship would mean that they would not have the opportunity to define themselves as siblings. The distance allowed her to close off possible social interaction, and thus stop the relationship from becoming more sibling-like.

Not everyone, however, expressed this anxiety about clear boundaries between themselves, the donor and the donor's family. Rather than seeing them as a threat, some families nurtured the connectedness that came with a known donor. Abigail and Jonathan, for example, cherished the connection they had with their donor and her whole family:

Abigail: We all have a lovely time together, don't we? When we all get together it's such fun . . . . Their children love [our son], don't they? . . . You know, lots of excitement when we all get together.
Jonathan: And he's excited by them. And we have photos of them around. Well, in his room he's got important people.
Abigail: In that frame.
Jonathan: And they're part of that; grandparents and everybody. (222)

The couple actively promoted the relationship between their son and his donor connections. Meeting up regularly, framing a photo of them as important people and displaying it in their son's bedroom became part of the family practices (Morgan, 1996) they engaged in to keep the relationship active. Interestingly, the donor and her partner had in turn offered a reciprocal connection by inviting Abigail and Jonathan to act as godparents for their own children, thus creating another connection across the families:

Jonathan: She had offered to be donor and when Abigail was pregnant... they asked us to be godparents to the children.

Abigail: That felt really good actually.... An acknowledgement of sort of common kin.

These two families were actively seeking, rather than guarding against, connectedness with one another.

Whether families sought a separation of kin or encouraged a social relationship to form, a relationship unfolded along the lines of relatedness that known donors bring. A common denominator for these families was therefore that they managed to coexist in a relationship with the donor (and his or her family) and that they would continue to do so as their child grew up.

Relationships, time and change

An additional aspect that was relevant in stories about known donor relationships was that relationships could shift and change over time and that it was impossible to imagine how they might unfold in the future. As we showed in Chapter 1, this aspect of relational life can bring challenges of particular kinds to the family of a donor conceived child. Angela and Samantha provided an arresting example of how relationships can evolve in the face of changing circumstances. Their story also illustrates how they, as the intended parents of a donor conceived child, managed the fact that radical changes were introduced in their family life. In this final section of this chapter, we recount their experience in some depth.

The couple had a son through donor insemination; Samantha had wanted a known donor and the couple approached a friend, Jason, who agreed to donate. The arrangement was such that he would not be involved as a father. Samantha became pregnant, and at that point Jason started to become interested and wanted more involvement, despite their previous agreement:

Samantha: When he came along and offered [to donate], his ideal role for him was 'I'll donate. I'll just be a friend of the family and I'll be Uncle Jason' and that was it. But as soon as I got pregnant, he wanted to come to the scan, and you can imagine the typical 'Oh'. And there was a connection.

Angela: And the 20 week scan just threw him, didn't it? (107)

Jason started to feel rather differently about the conceived child and during the pregnancy he suggested that he should be known as the father, rather than donor, thus seeking to be included in the family of the child. He also wanted to introduce the child to his own parents, who he wanted recognised as grandparents. Samantha and Angela had unexpectedly to contend with the idea of inviting into their family both an extra parent and an extra set of grandparents. This renegotiating of the family boundaries was not easy to accommodate. The relationships remained amicable, but Angela noted:

> Angela: At one point we really thought, 'Oh my God, it's just getting too much. Just leave us alone.' And I, I think more so than Samantha, felt, 'I don't want anyone else because I always said I want us to be the parents. I don't want a big communal family and joint decisions. I want us to be the parents, to live with our son, and that's the family unit.'

Then Jason's mother fell terminally ill. She had always wished for a grandchild, and she was overjoyed about the news of the baby. Due to her illness, the couple started to visit with the baby every week. By the time she died, the child had become the focus of both her and her husband's life. After her death, the baby started filling an important space in the life of the paternal grandfather:

> Samantha: Her passing away left a big hole for... the paternal granddad .... And that's been the basis of a real close relationship between them [him and our son].
> Angela: And he had to promise [the paternal grandmother] on her deathbed that he would really look after [our son]. In fact, after she died, it was what got him out of bed.

This grandfather had since become a very important figure in the little boy's life. He was closer to him than any of his other grandparents, and he saw this grandfather weekly. It was clear from our interview that this development was not altogether easy for Angela and Samantha to live with, although they accepted the situation.

> Angela: It is quite a big thing, you know, when [these grandparents] come [into your house] and you barely know them. It's still,

up to this day, this negotiation of paternal granddad wants us to be a complete part of his family, but we have no blood relation to him. And sometimes he oversteps the mark a little bit. You know, [he will say] 'Oh, you really ought to do this now,' and you think, 'Oh, hang on a second, who are you?'

Not all known donor relationships lead to this level of closeness, but what this story illustrates is how relationships can develop over time and the peculiar challenges that this brings in the context of donor conception. Much is at stake as the boundaries of families become more porous and as people who were strangers become relatives and make claims on the child. This case also shows how the known donor relationship not only concerns the parents and the donor, but also potentially involves others who make their own decisions about what the donor conceived child means to them. Parents (and donors) are not in control over how known donor relations evolve within these networks of donor kinship connections.

Conclusion

This chapter has explored donor relationships and how parents experience them after the birth of a child and as the children grow up. The unknown donor relationship has designed within it a clear sense of separation from the receiving family and connections are either completely severed or postponed until the child is an adult. However, our interviews show that the donor does not just vanish but continues to live on, in various shapes and forms, in the family. So although there is supposed to be no relationship during childhood, an imaginary relationship clearly exists for most receiving parents and, for some, the donor is present as a kind of ghost discernible in the child or lurking in the future. It is therefore possible to say that there are meaningful relationships that are ongoing through childhood with both unknown and known donors. Both raise issues that travel into the future with the child as he or she grows up.

It is the genetic relationship between the donor and the donor conceived child that frames these latent and/or unrealised connections. This is because the genetic connection cannot be fully ignored or transcended; it is culturally coded as meaningful and inscribed within systems of kinship. This means that there is forever an underlying, unresolved tension in the donor relation. The donor is not under-stood as a parent, nor as family, and yet the genetic contribution means the donor (and his or her relatives) can *potentially* claim to be connected. Properties of kinship and relationality are built into the donation and this is what emerges in different guises in the accounts of these parents. It emanates from questions about what a child is like, from the idea of 'donor siblings' and from the efforts to *not* know about potential kinship connections. It arises in the prolif-eration of kinship in known donor arrangements and frames these relationships. All these practices reflect and manage the same issue, namely the kinship connections that reside in the donation. There is a constant potential for the donor to fall into the kin category despite being positioned and conceptualised as non-kin. Families of donor conceived children have to manage this ambiguous place of the donor as part of their everyday family life.

7

(Not) One of Us: Genes and Belonging in Everyday Life

Introduction

> Erin: I'm 100 per cent her mum but I'm not the only person that made her. (217)

In this chapter we discuss the complex meaning of genetic connections in families of donor conceived children. Having a child of one's own is deeply framed by ideas about genetic relatedness, and we have already seen in Chapter 2 how very upsetting it can be for heterosexual couples to come to terms with the inability to conceive a child together and that the step to using donor gametes may be an extremely difficult one. Although donor conception is experienced as a more positive choice for lesbian couples, they nevertheless have to come to terms with the non-genetic links in their families and the genetic contribution of a donor. What makes donor conception so challenging for many couples is that the introduction of donor eggs or sperm into the family also introduces questions about whether and how they can claim that child as their own. It also raises questions about how the child can be viewed as a child of the family. The issue of genes and blood gives rise to a range of feelings in these families, because the donor conceived child is simultaneously perceived as a child 'of the family', while also being recognised as being different. As the title of this chapter implies, it is a child who is both 'one of us' and not. In this chapter we address the complex range of feelings that genetic connectedness gives rise to in families of donor conceived children. First, we address how families claim the donor conceived child as a child of their own and negotiate the presence of stranger genes. Thereafter we go on to explore the instances when genetic disruption and/or the donor genes come to the fore.

A child of our own

Parents and grandparents expressed the view that a donor conceived child born into their family was a child who belonged with them in a range of ways. They saw the child as theirs and yet to claim him or her as their own was not altogether straightforward. The child's different genetic ancestry could not be entirely ignored, and so families had to find ways of claiming the child as theirs while also taking account of the genetic donation. Four strategies emerged as particularly salient ways through which parents and grandparents negotiated claiming the donor conceived child. The first strategy was negotiating the meaning of pregnancy and bodily bonds. The second method was to deny that the genetic contribution of the donor would be of any particular significance. Third, family members emphasised social aspects of parenthood and family life over genetic ones. And fourth, families mapped family resemblances across non-genetic relationships as a way of creating an indisputable connection with the child.

The meaning of pregnancy and bodily bonds: Egg donation

Jacqueline: I was completely in favour of [egg donation]. Well, I mean, it's so much more your own child than adopting. That's what I said to [my daughter]. I said, 'You're going to feel it's yours, because you know, you've got a completely, you go through a completely normal pregnancy. Before you know where you are, you'll forget it's not all yours.' (Grandmother, heterosexual egg donation) (414)

The process of carrying a child to term fills an important cultural space, and we have already discussed how it links in with understandings and experiences of womanhood. Notwithstanding the fact that donation means using the genetic material of another man or woman, it affords women the experience of being pregnant and giving birth. Jacqueline (above) talks from a grandmother's perspective and she was typical in perceiving donation as preferable to adoption because it allowed the intended mother the experience of carrying the child. Pregnancy was attractive because it was conceptualised as making it possible for the woman to establish links with the foetus; links that bequeathed the woman more connection with the child. In Jacqueline's words, the pregnancy enabled a particular set of feelings to emerge; it would instil in the intended mother the feeling that it was more her child.

Shirley, the grandmother of an egg donor child, spoke in more depth of the bodily connection afforded through pregnancy:

> Shirley: Funnily enough my friends say, 'Oh, I can see [your daughter] in [your grandson] when she was that age.' Mmm, yes. And, you see, she has nurtured him. She's fed and nurtured him, there's got to be something of her in him although it's just not her egg, there's got to be a great deal of her in him. Nine months she's been feeding and nurturing him so part of her body and her fluids and everything else feeding him, got to be. (409)

Shirley interpreted comments made about family resemblances as evidence that her daughter's pregnancy had left traces in the grandson that were now becoming visible through his appearance. These traces are depicted in her account as laid down through the process of the child growing in the womb. The pregnancy is seen as a process through which the daughter has fed and nurtured the baby. Borrowing from the work of Monica Konrad, we might understand Shirley's way of making sense out of this process as a blood imaginary, a depiction of pregnancy as a process of providing 'blood food' (Konrad, 2005:155). If the genetic connection is culturally perceived as the substance of a kinship relation (Carsten, 2001; Strathern, 2005), then Shirley renegotiates the meaning of such bodily connections, substituting the genetic material with another kind of bodily connection, that of blood food. Genes and blood, which in conventional kinship thinking are conflated into one category, are separated out. This allows families of egg donor children to activate a line of kinship between mother and baby based in the body. Notwithstanding the stranger genes, the mother is, through this complex negotiation, to be found in the child. In this sense, the gestation inhabits the same cultural space as the genetic substance of the donated egg and can restore the connection that the donor egg disrupted.

By constructing pregnancy as a way for the mother to be present in the child, parents and grandparents were also able to negotiate the role of the donor's genes in the child. This was highlighted in Erin's account, in which she talks about why she preferred donor conception to adoption:

> Erin: I mean [donor conception] seemed like the next best option, it seemed like the closest that we could get to having our absolute own genetic child. I always kind of thought about it like... a bit of a pie chart really. So I've thought okay, let's say we are all half environment and half genetics and so when this baby pops out... half of its make-up is going to be from my husband so it's his environment, his involvement, his genes. And then it's going to be no genes from me so that's a quarter missing but it's going to be 75 per cent because it's going to be, you know, my environmental input. And then I thought to myself, well I've had this little baby growing inside me so maybe it would be a different genetic make-up, well it's come out differently because it's been carried by me, so I kind of added another kind of 10 per cent maybe, so I'm up to 85 per cent (laughter) so I mean, you know, so my pie chart's almost 100 per cent. (217)

As Marilyn Strathern (2005) argues, both social and biogenetic worlds of kinship make up tools for social living. Erin imaginatively draws on both relational (social) ways of relating and conceptual (biogenetic) ones to position her child in her family and that of her partner. She relates to a lay discourse about nature and nurture, which are imagined to contribute equally to the making and development of a child. But her account of conceptual kinship is distinctly different from conventional ideas of genetic knowledge. By separating out the meaning of genes from blood – describing herself as the blood parent – she negotiates the donor's contribution to the nature category in the nature/nurture binary. She means that the nature of the child has been altered by the experience of being carried by her, and this makes it possible for her to claim having contributed to the nature of the child. Additionally, she says she and her partner have shaped the baby fully through their nurturing. Through this reasoning the contribution of the donor is, in her mind, almost negligible. The underlying message here is that this means that she belongs with Erin. Pregnancy is thus perceived to compensate for the disruption of bodily connections that donation brings about.

Discounting the significance of genetic linkages

Phyllis: You see we don't think of him as that [donor conceived]. He's ours. (Non-genetic great-grandmother, heterosexual embryo donation) (412)

Betty: [We] just took [our grandson] as our own.... You know, from him being born, we just took it that he was ours (laughter). (Non-genetic grandmother, lesbian sperm donation) (314)

Phyllis was the great-grandmother of an embryo donation child, and Betty the mother of the lesbian non-birth mother of a donor conceived son. Both insisted that the disruption of genetic ties within their families was utterly insignificant, and they depicted genetic linkages as irrelevant to the creation of family belonging. These accounts are illustrative of the strategy that we refer to above as discounting the significance of the donor's contribution to claim the child.

It might be assumed that a strategy of discounting reflects a true indifference to donation and genetic linkages. However, we found that discounting practices were something that assisted families in containing the meaning of donor eggs within a social and cultural context where the idea of a 'proper family' (see Chapter 1) tends to be seen as synonymous with genetic kinship. Often these practices appeared in tandem with a very strong sensitivity to the perceived risks of not being recognised as the rightful family of the child. For example, Phyllis felt that the other residents in her retirement home would not be sympathetic to the use of embryo donation and so she kept it a well guarded secret. Similarly, Betty and her partner Richard were fully aware that their place as grandparents was precarious and were relieved when their daughter secured her status as a legal parent through adoption.

Discounting strategies could also take the form of minimising the genetic contribution of the donor. For example, Shirley had developed an elaborate idea of why a donated egg should be considered to be of minimal significance:

Shirley: I said to [my daughter], 'Well, you know, an egg, it's not like adoption where you're having the baby and giving the baby away so you're nurturing it for nine months. You're just giving an egg. And each month you have a number of eggs that just come away from your body so those eggs are not precious to you.' In fact, what I did say to her was, 'You go to the toilet and get rid of pooh that is no longer any use in your body and the egg is just the same. It comes each month and it, you just dispose of it. You're not attached to it in any way are you? It's not a baby and you never think, each month, these are potential babies....' [The donor] wasn't giving away something that was precious to her or significant to her, it was just meaningless. (One grandson, heterosexual egg donation) (409)

By focusing on what happens in women's bodies when eggs are not fertilised and constructing them as bodily waste, Shirley creates a narrative about eggs (and their genetic content) as meaningless. By developing this framework of thinking, she bypasses a discourse of how eggs and genetic links inform notions of kinship and belonging. Brenda, a mother of twins through egg donation, spoke in similar terms. She initially rejected the idea of egg donation, thinking that by accepting a donated egg she took another woman's children. However, by talking to a counsellor, she was able to reconceptualise the meaning of eggs:

Brenda: The counsellor made me see that I'm not taking a child from somebody, I'm taking, you know, a pinhead miniscule bit of data from somebody. (Mother of twins, heterosexual egg donation) (211)

So, rather than understanding this process of discounting as signalling indifference, we suggest that it indicates a way of managing donation, which is experienced as potentially problematic.

The importance of parenting

The third strategy by which families claimed a child as their own was by identifying the key essence of parenthood and defining it as a role based on social interaction rather than biogenetic linkages. Erin, for example, who renegotiated the meaning of genes and belonging, also spoke of how she saw motherhood as the outcome of social practices, relating this to the meaning of egg donation:

Erin: Becoming a mum, you know that there isn't anybody else who's [my daughter's] mum because it's the hours and hours and days and months and weeks and years of kind of love and time and energy and, you know, hard graft at times that you need to give to your child to raise it. To me it's become abundantly clear that that's what makes a mother and not the cell that starts it off so I don't have any problems with, you know, who is [my daughter's] mum. I'm 100 per cent her mum but I'm not the only person that made her, so it's a funny one. (217)

Erin focused on the social and interpersonal aspects of *doing* parenthood, and this helped her to negotiate what it meant to be a mother. She balanced her efforts in time and love invested in her daughter against the effort of the egg donor and asserted that by parenting her child she had come to realise that it is the everyday efforts of parenthood that makes a mother and not the genetic links through an egg. And so by drawing on and carefully emphasising the importance of social relationships and practices of care in forming kinship bonds and creating family life (Morgan, 1996; Strathern, 2005; Mason, 2008) she claimed her place as a proper mother. This also made it possible for her to announce that she was the mother, while also taking account of the donor's contribution.

The 'doing' of parenthood was also seen as important because it was understood to shape a child in unique and specific ways. Hannah, for example, had a granddaughter by egg donation and, in this case, the donor was a family member. Her daughter had conceived using gametes from Hannah's niece (on her brother's side). Hannah was immensely grateful to her niece and yet struggled with defining proper family boundaries and relationships following the donation. The donation was something she said she preferred 'not to think about too much'. By talking of parenthood as a practice which shapes a child in a unique way, she emphasised the importance of social parenting over genetic bonds and was thereby able to claim the child for her own family:

Hannah: Well I look at [my granddaughter] now and I see, you know, [my daughter] is her mother. She's going to be brought up with our ideals, she'll be educated in a way... I mean, [my daughter] has no television because she thinks it's much more important to read books and all that sort of thing. So I know she's going to be brought up in a very different way, probably, than she would have been brought up had she been with [my niece]. So I feel she's very much going to be ours. And I am a great believer in nurture. I suppose it's 50 per cent nurture, 50 per cent genes but I think that nurture's terribly important. And I mean, in a way, bringing up a child is what makes you closer to it. That's where the closeness comes from really, you know, not the genes so much. [My daughter] will do everything for this little mite. And as a family, we will be doing everything. So I feel as time goes on, she becomes more and more... Of course, she's is my daughter's husband's, it is his natural child as well, so I feel in many ways she's *not at all a stranger* in the family, if you know what I mean. So that gets better and better, actually, I have to say. (Emphasis added) (401)

Hannah clearly struggled with the significance of her niece's genetic contribution, and this kind of dilemma brings the question of belonging into sharp focus. She was seeking ways of thinking about the donation while also claiming the child for her daughter (and herself). Hannah suggested that the love, care and particular parenting style of her daughter and son-in-law meant that the child will develop in a way *which is unique for the family* and this would mean that, over time, she would become more theirs.

Creating family resemblances across non-genetic relations

Family resemblances play an important role in family life and are culturally coded as signifying genetic relatedness and a family bond (Mason, 2008; Marre and Bestard, 2009). So the tendency to imagine similar facial characteristics, or more fleeting things like a smile or a frown, or even talents and characteristics (such as a good singing voice or an optimistic demeanour) is now a well documented family practice. Thus, it is not surprising that these practices are often experienced as an issue of some sensitivity in families of donor conceived children where parents often worried about a lack of resemblance (Becker *et al.*, 2005; Nordqvist, 2010). But we found that, notwithstanding these sensitivities, family members often used resemblances as a way of conferring family relationships in the *absence* of genetic connections. Nancy, the non-genetic grandmother of two donor conceived children in a lesbian mother family, felt saddened by the fact that her grandchildren were not genetically related to herself but she took comfort in seeing that the children resembled members of her own family:

> Nancy: It's really okay, you know. I mean you like to see those little characteristics of family in the child. But if you don't, it's okay. You can still really pick them out anyway because everybody's the same. And you know, where I see temper here, I see my brother's temper in [my grandson], so it's the same thing. Yeah, I see brown eyes in [my granddaughter], my brown eyes, the same thing. So I mean you could make it work, it's no problem. (302)

Despite the lack of genetic connections between herself and her grandchildren, Nancy is able to see her own family reflected in the children. She is clearly keen to make such connections, suggesting that you can 'make it work' despite the lack of a genetic relationship. To her, the similarities she noted were significant because they allowed her to construct links between the children, herself and her family.

Far from feeling cautious about seeing family resemblances in their families, parents and grandparents of donor conceived children perceived and mapped resemblances across non-genetic family relationships. An example of this emerged in our interview with Jenny, who spoke at length of the similarities between herself and her daughter and how important it was that others recognised that likeness:

> Jenny: I think she looks like she's ours. I think she looks like Miranda's [partner] and like mine. Certainly my family have commented like, 'Oh my God, she really looked like you just now...'. And my sister will say, 'You used to do that when you were little'... (sighs)... I don't know, but I recognise that it's something that I foster and I recognise that... I take a small, you know, crumb and make a cake out of it.... I like it because she's my child. She's my child and I like the physical evidence of it, you know. (Lesbian mother, sperm donation) (121)

Mapping resemblances emerged as an important strategy that enabled parents and other family to claim connectedness with the donor conceived child. We also found that the ability to see likeness in the family filled an important function for some in terms of managing the child's donor origins.

> Joanne: I think if the character of the child links with the fam-
> ily, I don't think that it [genetic origin] matters that much, if
> you see what I mean. I think I would have been very hurt if
> [my grandson] he'd... either been very violent or something or
> other, you know, and that sort of thing.... He wouldn't have fit-
> ted in, [that] would have worried me somewhat I think. (Paternal
> grandmother, heterosexual egg donation) (408)

When asked about how 'fitting in' felt to her, she responded:

> Joanne: Well, I think it brings out the belonging if you know what
> I mean.
> Petra: Belonging to the family?
> Joanne: Belonging to the family, yes. I mean, okay you don't
> always look for red hair or if they're very good with their hands
> or something or other, but you know it's lovely to be able to say,
> even if it isn't true, 'Oh, he's just like his father' (laughter).

Resemblances play an important role in our cultural imagination about what ties families together and they operate as a way of sig-nalling family belonging (Strathern, 1995). As Signe Howell (2001) has argued in relation to adoptive families, we can understand fam-ily resemblances as a social currency that allows families to bring a non-genetically related child into a lifecourse which overlaps with their own. Joanne's account suggests that if a child resembles fam-ily members then it is easier to cope with 'stranger genes' because the family can still operate as normal. But equally, as Nancy above points out, even where there are no obvious resemblances it is per-fectly possible to act as if there were and thus integrate the child in the normal way.

Not one of us

Notwithstanding the rich and varied ways in which parents and grandparents claimed the donor conceived child as a member of their family, the issue of having a child who was in genetic terms a relative stranger was never fully forgotten. In this section we discuss some of the instances where families were reminded of a child not being fully theirs. In the first instance we explore the process through which families came to think of a child being different from others in the family. Ordinary, everyday struggles could become linked to ideas of genetic disconnectedness and this, almost inevitably, returns us to the significance of family resemblances. Finally, we address how many parents and grandparents continued to feel an ongoing sadness about a discontinued genetic line.

Seeing differences

Above we have shown the social importance that is attached to mapping likeness and similarities in families. But by the same token, we found that signs of a child being different in some ways raised questions about belonging and not-belonging. We discovered that one of the instances when parents and grandparents were reminded of the child's genetic origins was when she or he expressed something that did not seem to fit with the rest of the family; for example, having a specific talent or an interest that seemed foreign. This reminded them that the child was, in some sense, related to someone else.

> Betty: I mean, I often wonder what [the donor] looks like. . . . Like [our grandson] will do something and I think, I wonder if your father . . .
> Petra: Like what for example?
> Betty: Well, I mean, he's a very, very good swimmer, isn't [he]? You know, and I often wonder if his father was very sporty or . . .
> Richard: Yeah, he's into all the swimming, kickboxing, and all this sort of thing . . . .
> Betty: . . . [because his birth mother] she's not very sporty. (Non-genetic grandparents, lesbian sperm donation) (314)

Differences are of course present in every family, but it appears that when they occur in the family of a donor conceived child, the genetic donor would spring to mind and frame understandings of that difference. Many grandparents, in particular, spoke of being curious about what the donor had been like, based on how they saw a child developing.

We think it is important to acknowledge, however, that curiosity about a child's difference often sat alongside a complete acceptance of the child as a son, daughter or grandchild. Identifying difference did not signify rejection of the child. Sheila, a non-genetic grandmother of two children conceived using both donor eggs and donor sperm in a Spanish clinic, said the donor conception made no difference in terms of seeing the children as her grandchildren. And yet at the same time, their genetic origins did bring out questions for her:

> Sheila: Sometimes you think, 'Good Lord, what on earth's going on there? That's not Jill or Mike....' Well, they [both] like olives, none of ours ate olives. [These children] like olives. And I'm thinking, you know, is that something to do with a Spanish inheritance, a gene or something? I don't know. I'm fine about that, I think that's great. (407)

Everyday struggles

When family life felt like a struggle some parents would ask themselves if their endeavours were in some way caused by a lack of genetic relatedness with their children. Erin, for instance, found the first year of full time motherhood at times very difficult and this brought up questions about her ability to parent the child:

> Erin: I think that's really quite a difficult time [the first year], well it certainly was for me anyway because you are thrown into this kind of complete maelstrom and I think, with being the parent of a donor conceived child particularly, [...] I think if you're not the one who's got the genetic connection it's just an extra layer of things to try and kind of come to terms with and it's such a shame because you struggle and everybody struggles when they're a first-time parent but I think that it's difficult for a donor conceived child's parent.... There's a tiny little voice saying at the back of your head, 'Maybe it's because I'm not genetically related to this human being.' When they cry and you can't settle them and just nothing seems to work and you don't know what you're doing, you are in this kind of massive confusion and

it's very scary and it's very daunting. I think it's a shame really but you do have that. There are times when you know you're at your lowest ebb and you just think..., 'This baby knows that I'm not their genetic mum,' which is a load of old bollocks basically but at the time you do, you do kind of question it, you do find yourself thinking it. (217)

Whereas Erin was aware that parenthood is a difficult task for anyone, in her mind being a non-genetic parent of a donor conceived child added an extra layer of difficulty. The lack of genetic connection made her question herself as a parent, and her ability to meet her child's needs. Although it is clear from her account that she did not believe that there is any essential difference in being a genetic or non-genetic parent, at times of difficulty and vulnerability, when she was at her lowest ebb, questions about her connection to her daughter would niggle at the back of her mind.

We also found that a non-genetic parent could doubt their bond with their child and their own identity as a parent. For Trevor, a non-genetic father, the issue of sperm donation was always at the back of his mind and it became a greater concern when he struggled with parenthood. For him and his partner Monica, this was an ongoing issue. Trevor felt he had to compensate for his lack of connection by being a better father:

Trevor: You're constantly trying to make sure you are doing, [that] you are there and you are putting in the full effort possible.... You know I have to make sure that I put in the effort because, if I am missing something through the biological, I don't want it to be a problem.
Monica: I think you almost kind of overcompensate and put pressure on yourself and, in a kind of opposite way, I probably overcompensate about how I put the message of what a wonderful daddy [you are] across to [our daughter] (laughter). (213)

These accounts suggest that non-genetic parents can feel particularly vulnerable in their parenthood. Whereas the genetic parents in our sample did not appear to look for answers when they struggled with their children, non-genetic parents could doubt their ability to parent. For them, the missing genetic link translated into self-doubt and feelings of not being fully parents. This resonates with the point that Janet Carsten (2004) has made, that genetic kinship is culturally understood as a relationship that is given as opposed to an affinity that is made. What we might see emerging in these accounts is the pressure felt among non-genetic parents to make themselves into *proper* parents because they were unable to tap into a cultural understanding of their parenthood as simply given.

Similar concerns emerged in our interviews with grandparents who spoke of how a non-genetic relationship might raise difficult questions at times.

> Wendy: I honestly don't know whether it would have mattered to me or not [being a non-genetic grandparent]. I don't think it would, not in the baby stage it wouldn't have mattered. I think when it gets to the children stage, one tends to love one's own children and perhaps not everybody else's because, for whatever reason, children can be very irritating. So I think I can understand why there could be difficulties later on with grandparents that are not genetically connected because you haven't got that bond. I mean if it is your own, if you are genetically connected, I think you always feel a certain responsibility to how that child has turned out, you know. (Maternal grandmother, heterosexual sperm donation) (405)

Genetic kinship is often popularly understood as a fixed and non-elective kinship (Finch and Mason, 1993; Mason, 2008) and this belief appears to frame Wendy's account in which she suggests that the genetic family connection is more able to withstand the pressure of everyday family life. Genetic connectedness is perceived to provide something of a security blanket because embedded in that connection is the idea that grandparents have some responsibility for the ways in which new generations turn out (Mason *et al.*, 2007:692). Wendy suggests that non-genetic grandparents may not feel the same responsibility and would therefore also be less resilient in dealing with difficult children. This issue ties in with how genetic connectedness can play a central role in grandparents' acceptance of their grandchildren which came through with particular force in lesbian donor conception (see Chapter 3).

Family resemblances again

As we note above, one issue that brings donor origins to the fore are comments made about family resemblances. Whereas talk about resemblances for some families allowed them to negotiate a non-genetic family relationship, it was in other families experienced as a potentially negative and hurtful subject. This is illustrated by James's account. He was a non-genetic father who felt very sensitive about the use of donor sperm. He recalled one Christmas dinner when talk about resemblances had became a problem:

> James: Last Christmas, [my] parents were talking about how much Doodah was like Doodah and how much my brother's kids were like him, and what they were up to, and I went, 'Guys, can we just shut up.' Because that was really killing me. (laughter) It was Christmas dinner and so I had to, you know, I spoke out loud and just went, 'Look, you know, our kid's not going to be anything like me. This is really hurting. Let's move on.' And I think they needed to be a little bit more sensitive about that. Now, if they say, 'Oh, [your daughter's] got a mannerism like me,' then I can accommodate that. That's funny. But if they say, you know, 'Oh, look at her facial features,' I'm going to be, 'Come on, get real' (laughter). (203)

Comments about resemblances are culturally framed through genetic connectedness, and for James this meant that this dinner conversation reminded him too acutely of his lack of genetic connection to his daughter. This was also demonstrated in our interview with Sasha, who, although comfortable in her non-genetic motherhood, struggled with inferences made about resemblances between her partner Gemma and the children:

> Sasha: It drills home every time they [partner's parents] say it, that I'm not biologically connected and I suppose I'd just like them to be a bit more sensitive about it. (Two children, lesbian sperm donation) (114)

It might be assumed that the sensitivities about resemblances were only significant for the non-genetic parent in the couple but we found that they were an issue for both parents and they came to shape their relationship. For example, genetic mother Carrie found that genetic connectedness was something of a taboo subject between her and her partner Paul:

> Carrie: I don't [talk to Paul] because it's too hurtful I think – of the fact that... they're mine biologically and they're not his biologically. (Two children, heterosexual sperm donation) (208)

Carrie felt pleased that the children were genetically related to her, but felt that she could not enjoy that feeling as much as she would like:

> Carrie: I'd like people to say they look like me.... On the other hand, I don't want them to say that too often (laughs). For some reason they always seem to think they look like Paul. But yeah, I sometimes feel like I can't really kind of revel in that biological link... because I'd feel bad. [I feel like] he'd feel like I was rubbing it in.

The asymmetric genetic connectedness between parents could mean that being genetically related was connected to feelings of guilt and was felt to be a pleasure that had to be kept secret. This aspect of a relationship often had to be actively managed rather than ignored:

> Claudia: You know, there have been times when I've really struggled with... I was open at the beginning about how much I was gonna struggle with not being the biological parent and you've [Nina] worked really hard, haven't you, to make me feel like I'm as much the mum as Nina is really.
> Nina: We've just been gentle with each other, I think, haven't we? (Expecting a child, lesbian sperm donation) (116)

We also found that talk about family resemblances could be hurtful because it was perceived to upset the balance between the genetic and the non-genetic parent, and between the genetic and non-genetic side of the family.

> Erin: [M]y mother-in-law will say, 'Oh, you know, she looks just like Sinéad,' as in her own daughter, they'll see family

resemblances. And I know that they're never going to make a comment like that about me...I do think when they make a comment like that they're sort of claiming her for their own a little bit...like, 'Oh, you know, we can see our family in her.'...I sort of feel sad, a little bit sad because...I mean my family can't say that, you know, they can't say, 'Oh, he looks just like granddad,' or whatever. (217)

Sasha: I suppose [I mind Gemma's mother's comments about resemblances] because I also want them to have some kind of knowledge of my childhood and like every story is about Gemma, like every single thing that happens with the kids. (114)

Talk about family resemblances clearly taps straight into issues of genetic connectedness and disconnectedness and thus triggers potentially difficult feelings and uncertainties that can haunt the families of donor conceived children.

Ongoing feelings of loss and grief

In this final section we turn our attention to an aspect of genetic connectedness that played an underlying but ongoing part in the lives of families of donor conceived children, particularly in the context of heterosexual donor conception; namely the loss and grief associated with not having been able to conceive a child of 'one's own'. In Chapter 2 we wrote about the immense difficulties that heterosexual parents could experience in accepting donor conception as a route to parenthood. We found that this loss often remained after becoming parents. For Kevin, for example, this affected him greatly in the first year of his son's life:

Kevin: I kept getting sort of blindsided, emotionally and unexpectedly. Somebody would say something or I'd see something on the television and I'd be in pieces. And I didn't want that getting in the way of my relationship with [my son]. So I went and sought out a specialist in fertility counselling. (Two children, heterosexual sperm donation) (209)

Over the years, the moments when the sadness was acute would typically be fewer and less frequent. As a baby arrived and the practicalities of parenthood took over, the grief felt at infertility diagnoses would diminish. But our interviews with parents indicate that these feelings did not always disappear completely.

> Kevin: The therapist that I saw, the specialist in infertility that I still occasionally see, the way she refers to it is..., 'You've got a scar and it's gonna itch occasionally.' And she's absolutely right, it does. (209)

This sadness had a pervasive and ongoing presence in the lives of families. The non-genetic grandparents in the sample also spoke of a feeling of loss:

> Leonard: Well, one's naturally sorry that it's not one's own flesh and blood as it were. (One grandchild, heterosexual egg donation) (402)
>
> Alice: It's sad in a way because – not my bloodline but my husband's blood.... Well nearly all [his family] has gone. My son is one of the remaining [Winterbottoms] and there may be one in Australia and one in Canada but otherwise there's [no one], the line's gone. (Four grandchildren, heterosexual egg donation) (403)
>
> Frances: I do feel sad for [my daughter] in that there is nothing [in] the twins from her. (Two grandchildren, heterosexual egg donation) (413)

These ongoing feelings of sadness should not be understood to impinge on the delight and joy that parents and grandparents felt over the birth of the child. Rather these families were able to experience feelings of pleasure over having become parents (or grandparents) alongside their sadness over a lost genetic lineage. Thus, we found that families of donor conceived children lived with and managed the ongoing tension present in their lives between having become parents, but failing to do so in the way that they had hoped.

Conclusion

Genes and blood play a complex role in families of donor conceived children because such families negotiate claiming their child as their own in the presence of stranger genes. Negotiating the meaning of pregnancy, parenting practices, discounting the significance of genetic donation and mapping family resemblances across non-genetic relations are ways through which families find ways of claiming their child as their own and creating undeniable bonds of connectedness with him or her. On the other hand, various everyday instances remind parents and also grandparents of ways in which their family bond is also in question. For example, our interviews show how deeply families feel the disruption of genetic linkages, and how vulnerable people can feel as parents when they lack such links with their children. They also highlight how non-genetic family connections are perceived as more fragile. When family life is difficult, or when a child expresses a taste, talent or behaviour that does not seem to fit within the family, or which is not approved of, the missing genetic link emerges as a way of explaining these problems.

Parents' negotiations of genetic connectedness in claiming the donor conceived child as their own, as well as their ongoing feelings of vulnerability and loss, demonstrate how strongly genetic and bodily connectedness features in the contemporary cultural framework of what makes parents, family and kinship, and also what shapes ideas about family belonging. At times genetic connections in family life emerge as strong, given and fixed, whereas social ones surface as vulnerable and uncertain. The accounts and negotiations of genes and blood make sense only in a cultural context that defines genetic connections as real connections and where non-genetic family bonds are seen as less legitimate. Inevitably, parents of donor conceived children relate to the cultural significance ascribed to genes and blood and are consequently thrown into a process of claiming family bonds in a context where these are in question. In our final chapter we turn to the important issues of the cultural significance of genes and genetics.

8
Relative Strangers and the Paradoxes of Genetic Kinship

Zoe: I thought, actually no, if I got the chance, I would like to pass on my genes. (202)

Michelle: It sounds like I've got really bad genes; I haven't got bad genes at all. (118)

Nina: Because I think what we believe is that genetics isn't just about genes. Do you know what I mean? (116)

Norman: Yeah but we don't go – nobody goes around picking their parents by looking at their gene pool do they? (415)

Victoria: But put it like this: the way they interact with the children, you would never know there wasn't a genetic link. (212)

Linda: Yeah, we know that the genes work, as well. You know, the genes work well together. (111)

Theresa: But the thing is you don't know why a child develops like it does, because the genes are in it and I want an explanation of the genes. (303)

Judging from these quotations it would seem that the concept of the gene is now part of everyday thinking. The terms 'gene' or 'genetic' are routinely invoked when talking about family relationships, reproduction and children. These terms are in everyday use; in fact some now refer to the geneticisation of society because, in Western cultures, we seem to explain everything from aggression, intelligence, talent, appearance, taste, sexual orientation and health in terms of our genes (Haraway, 1997). But, if we look closely at these short quotations selected from the many remarks on genes made in the course of our interviews, it is possible to see that what genes are and what genes do is not terribly clear in people's thinking. The only elements that can be said to be a constant feature in these remarks are the thing-like quality of the gene and the gene's capacity to be very significant. This boils down to the idea that everyone has genes, everyone can share their genes with the next generation if they have children, and these genes matter. Beyond that point, understanding seems to blur and, as we showed in the previous chapter, there are very different kinds of consequences that flow from disparate beliefs about exactly how these genes work and how much they matter.

In this concluding chapter we will explore the question of how donor conceived families comprehend genetic connectedness in a context where there now *seems* to be a universal belief in the foundational quality of genes. We are not concerned with whether or not their knowledge of genes and genetics is scientifically correct; rather we are interested in what meanings are invested in the concept of genes and how much they matter in everyday relationships. In order to do this we start by considering the kinds of idioms that people use to express their kinship relationships and look at the shift in terminology from 'blood' to 'genes' which has occurred over the last 50 years. We will raise the question of whether the terminology of genes is simply a new form of packaging for longstanding ideas about biological relatedness and whether the concept of the gene has become a useful shorthand for depicting kinship. We will then situate these comments about genes and genetics in the broader context of the interviews we conducted, where we found that people held very complex and often quite contradictory views on the centrality of genes. Indeed, we discovered a profound paradox in the sense that it became clear to us that genes both matter a great deal and yet do not really matter at all. We suggest that it is important to read the everyday use of terms like 'genes' and 'genetics' carefully because such linguistic traits do not necessarily imply a commitment to genetic determinism in families.

From blood to genes

Steve Jones, the geneticist, has pointed to the way in which scientific ideas seep into everyday narratives and become part of informal (often confused) ways of understanding how biology works (1993, 1996). Of course this scientific discourse does not land on a blank canvas, so to speak, because local cultures always already have their own ways of comprehending issues of reproduction, inheritance and kinship which may come from tradition, religious teachings or a belief in myths and/or Mother Nature. What is more, as Jones is able to demonstrate, when we look back at early scientific discoveries or explanations it is possible to see very readily how science itself is infused with the traditions and cultures from which it emerges. Recognising the iteration between science and culture, indeed their profound interconnection, is hugely important in the process of understanding how new concepts like genes come to fill the public imagination.

One recent shift in scientific idioms has been the move away from the core concept of 'blood' to the now more ubiquitous concept of 'genes'. As Jones points out, the idea of inheritance, whether in human reproduction or livestock breeding, was based on the idea that the bloods of the father and mother were mixed together to produce the child. This idea was, and sometimes still is, reflected in common speech where, for example, ideas of the importance of the bloodline or of aristocratic (blue) blood were held to be very important. Equally significant could be ideas of bad blood which could enter into a family line and despoil resulting children, who would show traits of criminality or immorality. Concepts of racialised blood were significant too, as with the idea of miscegenation, through which white bloodlines could be contaminated or, conversely, through which black bloodlines could be improved. The tiniest drop of bad, mad or black/foreign blood in a family could be seen as disastrous. Although biologists started to give up on the idea of the significance of blood for inheritance in the early twentieth century it lived on in popular usage for a lot longer.

> Barbara: When I was a child, I had a friend who was adopted and my father found out in some way. She only lived up the road and he flatly refused to have her in the house....He said, 'I'm not having bad blood in the house.' And it was a generational thing, just after the war. It was shameful, out of wedlock pregnancy was shameful, you know, and the idea was that you'd got bad genes, as it were. (406)

Barbara is talking about social attitudes in England around 1950 or 1960 and in this case her father's belief, not fully articulated in this short extract, was that an adopted child would have originally been illegitimate and therefore the product of immoral parents who would have passed the contamination down the line. A respectable household would therefore guard itself against any ensuing social contamination by barring its doors against the child.

Ideas of bad blood now seem faintly quaint or even highly prejudiced to modern ears and it is rare to hear of people commonly speaking in these terms. In our interviews people rarely referred to blood in terms of inheritance or in relation to the idea of the bloodline and those who did were often the older generation or the older generation speaking of past attitudes. As Jones has argued,

> 'Blood feuds, blood brothers, blue blood, cold blood, bad blood' – all have shifted from the orbit of science into that of metaphor. But change the language a little, replace 'blood' with 'gene' and suddenly we are in the modern world. There is a new era of belief in the power of biology and a new fear of what we may find out about ourselves.
>
> (1996:4)

Of course the word 'gene' did not replace the term 'blood' overnight; as the quotation from Barbara above implies, there can still be a slippage between the two. It is interesting to see how she sought to explain the terminology of blood by bringing it *up to date* with a reference to genes. So the translation of blood into genes was a gradual process starting in the early twentieth century with the reappraisal of Mendel's work on the inheritance of traits across generations. The rise of the field of genetics has been mapped by biologists like Jones (above), Steven Rose (1997) and more recently Nessa Carey (2012). As Rose has pointed out, each recent discovery on the way has been presented in the media in a wildly exaggerated fashion, not only presenting individual genes as causing complex social behaviours or personality traits in a direct way but presenting gene therapy as the way to end behaviours such as violence, drug addiction, cancer, mental distress, obesity and even homosexuality. The idea appears to have been planted in the public imagination that genes determine all significant attributes in a person, from which it follows that it is sensible to be cautious about which genes you allow into your family gene pool. The 28 May 2013 issue of *BioNews*, a weekly electronic newsletter which carries up-to-date information on developments in policy and research in biogenetics, carried three articles on the links between genes and illness or depression. One announced a new genetic testing programme for cancer risk, a second covered the story of the first preventative prostatectomy in the UK and the third was a story about epigenetics (which we explain below) and post-natal depression. These stories (which were also reported in the national press) followed a week of international coverage in May 2013 of the actor Angelina Jolie's preventative double mastectomy, performed because she carries a gene associated with breast cancer. There is little surprise therefore that while ideas of bad blood are now seen as in bad taste or ignorant ramblings, ideas of bad or faulty genes hold a more plausible place in everyday discourses on inheritance.

It is not hard to agree with Jones that the old-fashioned term 'blood' has given way to a modern term like 'genes', but they are not entirely synonymous. One significant difference is that it is possible for a person to see blood, to touch it and to understand how it circulates in the body. It is a thick material fluid. But genes cannot be seen (other than in a laboratory) and how they work is much more mystifying (to scientists as well as lay people). If blood was accorded magical qualities in the past, then arguably genes are much more prone to this kind of treatment since only a few highly educated people can actually explain what they are and how they work. That is not to say that many have not tried and Richard Dawkins (1976), for example, in his mission to improve the public understanding of science, is foremost amongst them. However, what becomes immediately apparent in the work of all scientists who try to popularise such complex ideas is that they rely heavily on the workings of metaphor. Precisely because the science of genetics is incredibly hard for lay persons to grasp, all popular representations of the issues rely on metaphor to translate abstract concepts into culturally meaningful terms. This is what Dawkins has done with his idea of the selfish gene, what the *Daily Mail* did with the idea of the gay gene (Rose, 1997:275) and what has happened more generally to describe our genes as the blueprint for human life. As Rose points out:

> It is hard to know which had more impact on the future directions of biology – the determination of the role of DNA in protein

synthesis, or the organizing power of the metaphor within which it was framed.

(1997:120)

The notion of the metaphor is also alluded to by Jones in the above quotation, where he implies that as ideas slip out of the scientific laboratory they take the shape of metaphors. Of course, which metaphor is used and which one becomes more fixed in the imagination is incredibly important, as metaphors shape understandings of what genes are and how they work. So the idea of the selfish gene can frame a particular understanding of why individuals behave in the ways that they do; it also gives a huge significance to the single gene as if each one has its own drivers and power to determine outcomes alone. The idea of genes as a blueprint also gives genes an extraordinary power to determine outcomes while at the same time the genes themselves appear fixed, rigid and immutable. Increasingly the metaphor used to capture the concept of genes is the idea of a set of instructions or even simply information which is open to interpretation and influence by environmental factors. *BioNews*, for example, offers a helpful online glossary of terms and genes are there described there as 'an inherited instruction that tells the body how to make proteins'. And the anthropologist Carles Salazar uses a similar metaphor:

> To share genes does not mean to share any natural substance but to share information, 'intangible, non-material information'.
>
> (Salazar, 2009:181)

More recently Carey (2012) has changed the metaphor and argues that the genetic code should be understood to be a 'script' which is open to interpretation and different readings. Hence, she likens the genetic code to a script or play which, if written by Shakespeare, would be of high quality but which could be spoilt by poor acting or meagre direction. Alternatively, she points out, the script itself may be of inferior quality but salvaged by good acting and splendid direction. In her metaphor the gene is not an isolated, fixed entity but a malleable, interactive flow whose precise direction cannot be predicted in advance.

Emily Martin (2001) has traced the ways in which the cultural metaphors used to provide popular understandings of the working of the human body reflect dominant models of the workings of wider society. Hence she describes the rise of the idea of the body as a machine which could break down and fail to function properly. Such a metaphor, she argues, is closely linked to everyday understandings of industrial machinery and so it was a metaphor which 'worked' for a highly industrialised culture. Her interest was in women's understandings of their own bodies and she notes how, in the US, where she carried out the research, social class was also very significant in the ways in which girls explained menstruation to her. Thus middle-class, more educated girls described the cycle of menstruation in mechanical terms as one of preparation, failure and the production of waste product while the working-class, less educated girls used more biblical metaphors about 'the curse' or about menstruation as a rite of passage towards becoming a woman. More recently Mary Midgley (2010) has carried out a similar analysis of Dawkins' idea of the selfish gene, arguing that this metaphor grabbed the public imagination because of the political context in which it was published, namely extreme individualism promoted originally by the Thatcher government but continued by subsequent governments of various hues. These sorts of arguments suggest strongly that the metaphors selected by scientists are not random but already have their genesis in dominant social conditions and, for the same reason, we can see why the most contemporary manifestation of the gene metaphor is one based on notions of 'information' or 'codes'. In a digital, computer age such metaphors are readily understood and assimilated.

Kinship and relatedness

In Chapter 7 we explored in detail how the parents and grandparents we interviewed coped with genetic relatedness and unrelatedness in their everyday lives. As we suggested, in many ways the absence of genetic links has become the elephant in the room which has to be negotiated regularly and which at times seems to inflate to unreasonably large proportions. Families with donor conceived children, like adoptive families before them, are at the forefront of a modern debate about the conflicting significance of nature versus nurture. They seem regularly obliged to bring out the metaphorical weighing scales in order to work out which of these is more critical yet, even if parents feel they have achieved an equilibrium, inevitably a relative, neighbour or even complete stranger can tip the balance with a mundane remark. It is also very hard for contemporary parents to forget the possible consequences of genetic inheritance when it is on the news so regularly, forcing them to wonder whether their child has an invisible 'faulty' or problem gene.

> Cathryn: [My mother] still had a lot of kind of very dated ideas about well, you know, 'What if [the egg donor] is a criminal? You know, then you've got criminal genes in your family.' (201)

Parents and grandparents of donor conceived children may experience themselves as occupying a rather exposed position, socially speaking, because they seem to be required to shoulder the responsibility of sorting out contemporary, cultural expectations about genetic relatedness. Theirs is not a theoretical interest in the topic; they have to answer difficult questions even if the queries are posed only in their own minds or in private. Increasingly insistent demands that these parents should be entirely transparent about donor conception further isolate them with a private dilemma to solve – as if it was solely the couples who needed gamete donation who gave rise to this new social problem. One might be forgiven for imagining that before gamete donation came along, kinship was a straightforward matter where everybody knew who their biogenetic relatives were and that family life was solely based on this precise, and correct, information. Clearly the history of adoption which we discuss briefly in Chapter 1 gives the lie to this proposition, but also, as many students of kinship have shown, family life and relatedness have rarely been this simple (Carsten, 2004). Take for example the history of illegitimacy and paternity in England (Smart, 1987; Adair, 1996; Laslett, 2000). It was only in 1987 that the Family Law Reform Act moved to abolish the exceptional status of illegitimacy. Prior to that time, unmarried fathers were not regarded as legal fathers unless they married the mother of their child. It was the legal contract of marriage which created the recognition of fatherhood and not the biological connection. This lack of recognised connection between a biological but unmarried father and his child dates back to Victorian Poor Laws and although in some circumstances such a man could be obliged to pay towards the upkeep of his bastard children, typically the full responsibility fell on the shoulders of the mother. The converse of this situation was revealed in the legal position of all children born into wedlock because it was assumed that such children were always the biological children of their mother's husband, sometimes in the face of evidence to the contrary. English family law therefore did not follow rules of biological kinship, and regulations governing paternity were shaped in the interests of property transmission and in support of religious teachings on the immorality of bearing children outside wedlock. Moreover, as Carsten and other anthropologists have shown, kinship in other cultures is not directly based on biology – let alone genetics – with matters of religion, nurture or custom and practice determining who is related to whom. As both Carsten and Jeanette Edwards (2014) have shown, even in some modern, Westernised societies like Israel, kinship is determined by Orthodox religion not genetics. Thus in cases of egg donation where the egg is 'Jewish' and the sperm 'non-Jewish', the donor is erased entirely and children born into different families from the same donor's sperm are not regarded as (half) sibling.

Janet Finch (1989) has added further levels of complexity to this picture with her work on family obligations. She argues that in the UK, notwithstanding the legal or social position of members of a kinship network, public policy can operate a separate (but related) set of practices which create different kinds of connections between those who are genetically related and those who are not. Rules governing welfare benefits, for example, have sometimes been quite unconcerned with biological relatedness and have imposed, on men who cohabit with women who have children by another man, financial responsibilities to support those children until they reach adulthood. The creation of the concept of 'the child of the family' was a way of blurring distinctions between genetic and non-genetic children when it came to financial support. Finch also points to the concept of the 'liable relative', which was a device used to find biological kin to assume responsibilities above and beyond those normally anticipated as a duty of kinship. So while English law may offer some clarity about kinship and non-kinship, Finch shows clearly that the implementation of public policy may work with a different set of ideas about relatedness. Finch then draws our attention to yet another dimension of this contradictory picture which is the existence of what anthropologists refer to as 'local moralities'. At different times and in different places, a local morality might insist that an unmarried father takes responsibility for his illegitimate children, or it might expect adult daughters to leave employment to care for their aged parents, or it might assume that on divorce the children of a marriage rarely see their biological father again. Thus trying to trace how kinship works in practice is extraordinarily difficult (Finch and Mason, 1993) and it becomes clear that although there may be societal rules of kinship that one can discern, how people actually live their lives and what they think about kin can be much more fluid.

Carsten, for example, describes the ways in which it is common for people to pick and choose which kin they will relate to. Referring to English kinship, she points to the ways in which some kin are gently cut adrift, with the connection becoming little more than an exchange of Christmas cards and sometimes not even that. Moreover more distant kin may be favoured over closer kin so that, for example, a cousin may be kept closer than a sister, or an aunt closer than a mother. Earlier in the book we referred to this practice as 'de-kinning' because this captures the idea that we can actually choose our kin, in the sense that we need have nothing to do with those whose interests we do not share or who we simply do not like. The converse of this is, of course, the practice of kinning, through which family friends can become aunts or uncles to children, or the parents of a step-parent might become honorary grandparents (Howell, 2003). Anthropologists have also drawn attention to the importance of sharing houses and sharing food. Carsten argues that some of our most powerful childhood memories are embedded in the house (or home) we lived in as children. Thinking about different rooms such as kitchens or the place of the TV in the sitting room can conjure up strong feelings of connectedness (even if some are negative). She argues that family rituals (e.g. bath nights, storytelling at bedtime, Sunday breakfasts) can give rise to a very clear sense of kinship. In this we can see kinship being built up rather than being simply given through genetic connection. Edwards (2000) adopts a similar approach and has coined the term 'born and bred' kinship which was an idea that arose from her fieldwork in a small town in the north of England in the 1990s. She argues:

> My own interest...is in a society which mobilizes a distinction between the biological and the social, and which includes both in its delineation of relatedness. Rather than being *based* on the biological, however, the kinship on which I focus requires both

the biological and the social: it emerges from an interplay between the two, rather than from the social elaboration of natural facts.

(2000:28 emphasis in original)

In this passage Edwards invites us to go beyond the either/or of nature and nurture, and even to go beyond the idea that nature is a given upon which culture acts or plays out its role. Her focus on an interplay or iteration between the two is, we argue, an essential tool with which to understand the contemporary situation of donor conceived families. To explain what is meant by this interplay between the biological and the social, the role of food in the family provides a useful illustration. Feeding an infant may be regarded as the most basic act of nurture, as it is accompanied by physical and emotional closeness. But feeding also builds the child and, as Cathrine Degnen (2009) has shown, in Western cultures there is a strong belief that you are what you eat. Feeding a small child lots of crisps and chocolate might be understood to be an act of love and benevolent indulgence, but we also know that the child's body will grow and develop in specific ways as a consequence. Indeed their eating habits may be set for life giving rise to later illnesses or susceptibility to disease. The converse is telling as well; if a child will only eat jelly, which of course lacks essential nutrients, proteins and fibres, then the nurture side of the equation can become highly strained, making relationships difficult. Mealtimes can become a war zone leading to eating disorders and failure to thrive properly. Feeding is therefore all about nurture and incorporating children into kinship through the bonding that accompanies it, but it also has physical and bodily consequences. Degnen goes one step further in her analysis; she argues:

> First, feeding and eating are involved in the reproduction of social relationships, particularly family relationships. Secondly, cultural understandings of the role of food in the making of persons intersect with parental responsibilities in making *one's own kind of person.*

> (2009:46 emphasis added)

Here she is suggesting that through food mothers (typically) do not simply sustain a child's body and encourage it to grow, but that through specific choices of food and its whole organisation in terms of cooking, presentation, rules of consumption and so on, parents produce a child who mirrors the family's values and embodies their principles. There is a growing together through the sharing of the substance of food and this constitutes a most significant kinship practice. Returning to Edwards' point about the iteration between the social and the biological we can see, through this example, how difficult it is to slide a (metaphorical) cigarette paper between nature and nurture. The two fields work together creating different, even unique, combinations which suggests that adherence to a simplistic genetic determinism is increasingly fruitless. These studies therefore complicate kinship and it is important to hold this picture in mind when starting to understand the impact of the new genetics on kinship thinking.

Genetic thinking and kinship thinking

It can be argued that the rise of epigenetics (Carey, 2012) now suggests that biologists and geneticists are increasingly aware that genes do not tell the whole story of human life and relatedness, notwithstanding early enthusiasm about decoding the human genome. As Carey argues:

> When scientists talk about epigenetics they are referring to all the cases where the genetic code alone isn't enough to describe what's happening – there must be something else going on as well. [...] In [the molecular] model epigenetics can be defined as the set of modifications to our genetic material that change the ways genes are switched on or off, but which don't alter the genes themselves.
>
> (2012:6–7)

Of course, biologists like Steven Rose have long argued this case and have mounted arguments against genetic determinism (or its previous formulation as biological determinism) as being far too simplistic (Rose *et al.*, 1984; 1997). Together with Hilary Rose, he outlines the career of genetic and eugenic thinking in Europe over the twentieth century (Rose and Rose, 2012) and, although they document the inexorable rise of genetic thinking, as well as the Promethean promise implicit in mapping the human genome, they also note how the new genetics have failed to live up to early assertions about curing disease and eradicating disabling conditions. With the exception of single-gene disorders they note that all other attempts have foundered on the problem of complexity:

> That nothing turned out to be quite so simple came as no surprise to those unhappy with genocentrism. What the HGP [Human Genome Project] and the biobanks have revealed is a degree of biological complexity long suspected by less reductionist biologists but to which the sequencers and their backers, in their enthusiastic and single-minded pursuit, had turned a blind eye .... the completion of the sequencing of the human genome has produced a list of parts with no instruction book on how to put them together.
>
> (2012:281)

It may be possible to argue that the pioneering promise that genes could answer all our social and medical problems is now recognised as a chimera and there is a certain cooling of the early enthusiasms.

The question is, however, what has this crescendo of enthusiasm for all things genetic meant for everyday kinship thinking? We have argued above that, culturally speaking, ideas about genes are inevitably expressed in terms of metaphors and that recently these metaphors have shifted from ideas of fixed immutable blueprints to more flexible and malleable ideas of information or scripts. Of course, this does not mean that the popular media has caught up with the new terminology and, in turn, everyday thinking may still reflect the early hype surrounding the promise that genes could unlock the mysteries of inheritance. While there may be some truth in this cultural lag hypothesis (as some of the quotations at the start of this chapter *might* imply) we reject the idea that parents and grandparents slavishly but slowly follow where the scientists lead. As we point out above, scientific metaphors and messages, no matter how compelling, do not write themselves onto blank slates. If they did no one would smoke cigarettes, no one would binge drink and everyone would eat plenty of fresh vegetables or fruit. In the field of kinship such scientific messages have to contend with common sense, traditional beliefs, religious beliefs and scepticism as well as the everyday practices of kinship we have discussed above.

In order to explore the relationships between genetic thinking and kinship thinking we take three examples of the things that parents have said to us in their musings about relatedness. We have selected these because they reveal the complexity of their thinking and in particular how understandings (even misunderstandings) about how genes work are never unmediated by the cultural. In the first extract from Brenda (who is mentioned in the previous chapter) she is explaining how she came to terms with receiving an egg from a donor. We quote her at length because it is only when you can see the longer narrative that the complexities become apparent:

> Brenda: I thought, when we finally agreed to do it, I didn't feel the baby would be mine. I felt I would be taking a baby from somebody else. I felt very strongly about that.... It was a very odd feeling, you know, to be using someone's eggs. And I saw these eggs as children, I didn't see them as just eggs, as bits of tissue, I actually saw them as real children which is quite... I think it's quite a normal way to look at it when you first start thinking about it. And we did have counselling, we had to have counselling before our first donor egg treatment. And the counsellor made me see, you know, that I'm not taking a child from somebody, I'm taking a pinhead miniscule bit of data from somebody. And, oh no, those girls are mine absolutely (laughs). God, oh yes! I know that, you know, I grew them, without me they wouldn't even be here. (211)

In this account we can see what might be termed common-sense or even traditional thinking coming up against a more scientific narrative about the meaning of gametes. Brenda saw eggs as babies and, as she acknowledged, she is not alone in that. Indeed the whole anti-abortion lobby and much Christian thinking would roughly accord with this way of understanding gametes. She is encouraged to shift her thinking away from the idea of the egg as a virtually formed being to adopt the idea that these gametes are tiny bits of tissue. Tissue carries a very different set of meanings when compared with eggs, of course. But then later she shifts to the terminology of data in line with the metaphor of computer codes, data and information. Her understanding has apparently been reframed by the scientific discourse encountered at the clinic. But then she moves on to say unequivocally that her daughters are hers because she 'grew them'. She switches back into a more homely, almost horticultural metaphor which suggests that the clinching argument was her own fundamental bodily contribution to the growing of the babies. We found that other mothers who had had egg donation relied equally heavily on the huge significance of the embodied experience of gestation. In Chapter 7 we discussed how this can be seen as a process of minimising worries about stranger genes, but here we push that argument forward slightly to suggest that this kind of thinking, revealed in the slippage between very different explanatory metaphors, is commonplace when people seek to explain family relationships. They dip into a reservoir of ideas, many of which have competing epistemologies, in order to frame complex, abstract ideas about kinship. Brenda is not confused, nor does she slip from 'correct' scientific terminology back into 'misguided' common sense; rather she is deploying different aspects of available narrative explanations in order to cover the range of things she feels and experiences. She uses different metaphors to explain different aspects of the work of creating kinship.

Our next example concerns a story told to us by Cathryn about a close friend who was adopted as a baby. She uses this story as an analogy to make sense of the kinds of issues she is facing, having had a child by egg donation. She acknowledges that adoption is not the same as donor conception but she sees similarity in some of the core issues:

> Cathryn: Well, I know [James] who's our friend who's [our daughter's] godfather, he found his birth mother. He was adopted at six weeks old, and it's not the same, being adopted, it's not, I know it's not the same and there's a whole different set of issues. But he is probably more interested in his biological family history than he is in his adopted family history although he has closer relationships with his adopted family, and is [much] more tied to them but it – there's a different element which is I think to do with genetics and history and something very primal that ... (201)

In this extract there are a number of concepts at work. Firstly James is described as being more interested in his biological than his adoptive family history, but this is then contrasted with the statement that he is much closer to, and more tied to, his adoptive family. From this it would seem that James feels close to and loves his adoptive parents and he feels all the usual ties of kinship with them. He has an emotional interest in his adoptive family but he has an intellectual interest in his biological family. This account gives the impression that James is not particularly interested in relating to his actual biological kin; he is more interested in the abstract concept of lineage. Yet Cathryn reads a lot into this scholarly interest, seeing it as arising from (1) genetics, (2) history and (3) something primal. She does not elaborate on what the link between his interest and these three elements is but leaves her audience to surmise. Genetics comes first in her list, suggesting that genetic links carry both cultural and personal significance in some way. This is, of course, a very typical understanding of genetics. Then there is history, which suggests that knowing the biography of one's family or kin provides a sense of roots. The idea of roots was something that Edwards found to be a strong theme in Bacup, where she carried out her fieldwork:

> Roots connect places, persons, and pasts. In popular usage, one's roots refer to both family of origin and attachment to place.... 'Everybody needs roots,' I was told by one man, 'these children do as well.' Not knowing one's roots means, as one woman put it, 'having no real beginnings, no family and no ancestors'.
>
> (2000:229)

Edwards argues that donor parents, like adoptive parents in his case, are seen as being unable to offer a child a link to his or her whole past, his or her whole inheritance. However, what this story and also Edwards' research shows is that this idea of roots predates our contemporary fixation with genes. Thus a modern concept is translated through very old idioms.

The final concept in Cathryn's account is her reference to something primal. She does not finish this sentence but leaves it hanging as if she cannot quite pin down the thing she is trying to grasp. By primal she seems to mean something primitive, something buried in nature and also something beyond rational grasp. The primal seems to pre-date explanation and therefore cannot be elucidated; it just is. Cathryn's account therefore weaves together several different kinds of ideas as she works to make sense of her friend's actions and feelings. One idea is the contemporary halo of meanings around genetics, the second is a much older, more traditional concept of roots, and the third is rather mystical. Cathryn, like Brenda above, is operating as an everyday philosopher, piecing together elements of explanations to justify or clarify behaviour which is being played out on novel moral terrain.

Our last example is a brief comment that came from Carrie, whose husband was azoospermic. He had great difficulty coming to terms with his infertility and was initially reluctant to agree to sperm donation. However, at one stage he tried to persuade Carrie that, if there was going to be donated sperm, it should come from his brother because this would retain his (and his family's) genetic connection:

> Carrie: But then it almost seemed to me disloyal to conceive a child with his brother and it was like something out of Shakespeare. I just didn't like it you know. And, you know, I think obviously I didn't have to go and have sex with him or anything but Paul's argument was purely a typical man, 'Well that's the only way of getting some of my genes into this baby.' (208)

In this brief account we can see the ways in which gametes and genes can be evocative of two very different registers of meaning. For Carrie the idea of making a baby with her brother-in-law's gametes was a mixture of adultery (disloyalty), incipient tragedy (Shakespearean) and simply morally repugnant. Although it is possible to argue that a sperm is just a small amount of tissue or data (as with Brenda above), it certainly did not seem that way to Carrie. This sperm came loaded with meanings, mostly derived from quasi-religious teachings and an everyday moral calculus. She drew on traditional ideas of kinship and consanguinity in her thinking, and was unmoved by the genetic argument. Her reference to Shakespeare is also fascinating because it invokes ideas about outmoded codes of conduct, looming misfortune, adultery and an inappropriate closeness between brothers at the expense of a wife. For Paul, of course, it appears that it meant none of these things. By Carrie's account it was for him simply a rational way of ensuring genetic continuity and this goal was more important than any subsidiary emotions or objections. For Paul the genes were paramount, while for Carrie it was the nature and quality of relationships that mattered most. Carrie put these differences down to disparate, gendered sensibilities but we can also see that they are both drawing on equally current and persuasive discourses of the sort that abound in this field. In the end Carrie persuaded Paul of her views and they used an unknown, unrelated donor because his gametes were less contaminated with potent cultural meanings. In this very short story it is possible to see clearly how genetic thinking entwines with everyday kinship thinking and, in this specific encounter, the genes certainly do not triumph. It is therefore possible to argue that while the everyday language of family life now seems to give prominence to ideas of genetic connectedness, more complex and customary beliefs about kinship relatedness may not necessarily have changed very much.

Conclusions: Paradoxes of kinship

In the three stories that we have recounted above we can see the workings of kinship thinking. In cases of donor conception parents and grandparents are typically required to rehearse their thinking 'out loud' because they are pushed into a kind of limelight as they are constructing families in new ways. They need to find justifications, reasons and explanations for things that the majority of families can take for granted or can leave lurking in a kind of subterranean place which need not be disturbed. Parents who know (or think they know) that their children are genetic kin can shrug off many questions or doubts such as to why a child has temper tantrums, why they are musical, why they are slow learners and so on. They may not have adequate answers but they are likely to feel that the source of such behaviour could be traced to – or put down to – a known family background. With donor conceived children there is an apparent mystery, a kind of black hole made all the more significant by the modern emphasis on the foundational nature of genes. On the face of it, almost all of the parents in our study thought that genes were highly significant yet we found, like many others[1] before us, that kinship thinking was far more complicated than this. We found a paradox in that at times *real* kinship seemed to be imagined entirely in terms of genetic connection, while at other times genes were insignificant and subordinate to what *really* mattered in the doing of kinship. In her analysis of assisted reproduction and adoption,

Carsten argues that accounts people give ultimately have little to do with genetics 'although they apparently rely on sophisticated genetic arguments' (2004:179). She goes on to state:

> All of these scenarios involve participants deploying genetic arguments in a highly visible manner. But the results of these articulations show no retreat to a simplified and geneticized reading of kinship. Instead, we have seen how those concerned are able to achieve a complex 'choreography' between social and biological factors.
>
> (2004:179)

The parents and grandparents in our study also achieved a complex choreography between competing narratives and truths of kinship. Their reasonings were mobile and flexible; they changed according to the specific issue that they were addressing. They were very adept in combining the apparently unblendable into accounts which sustained their connection with the children they were raising who were not fully their genetic kin. Different parents created different combinations and some clearly found it extremely hard to resist a kind of genetic determinism, but the foundation of the kinship they were establishing was the raising, nurturing, sheltering and loving of their children.

In this book we have attempted to explore these experiences of having donor conceived children as fully as possible and we have not forgotten that parents live in a web of connections with wider kin and networks of friends. We have argued that these parents and grandparents, whether intentionally or not, have become a part of the contemporary process of redefining kinship. Their situation is special because they are (reluctant) pioneers and many were not necessarily prepared for the relational, practical and ethical challenges that their new form of parenthood would bring. Indeed, how could they be? They were all in a kind of cultural crucible in which elements of tradition, convention, inheritance, genetics, care and relationships mingled in different ways. All of our parents and grandparents wanted to 'do the proper thing' (Finch and Mason, 1993) in relation to their children and kin; it is just that it was not always clear what this was. This is why we discovered that telling children about their genetic origins was so difficult for almost all the parents, even those most ardently committed to doing so. It also explains why the different generations did not always share the same views and why different genders could experience things so diversely. The possible repositioning of the donor as potential kin was also something new that these parents had to contend with. This process is most visible with lesbian parents, but it is nudging its way into the lives of heterosexual parents too. Parents who received a tiny scrap of tissue or a mere cell (as framed by medical discourse) clearly found the idea that their child had another mother/father and other sibling (as framed by genetic thinking) when they thought they were creating their own family (as framed by kinship thinking) were obviously in an ethically and culturally complex position.

While we have argued that the parents in our study can be seen as being in a kind of involuntary cultural vanguard regarding the redefinition of contemporary kinship, it is also important to remember the specialness of our sample. Most of the parents we interviewed had pre-school children so they were in the midst of the process of disclosing to children their genetic origins. This means that they were quite fixated on the issues but it is quite probable that this preoccupation will change over time as the issues become subsidiary to other life events like schooling and examinations, friendships, going on to university and so on. Ideas about the importance of genetics might well wane as the children grow older or if, as a society, we become less obsessed with the significance of genes. In one or two decades the so-called geneticisation of society may reverse and nurture may seem more important again. Alternatively, by then we may have developed synthetic gametes or even acceptable forms of cloning, such that gamete donation from strangers or relatives becomes unnecessary. The experiences we have captured in this book are therefore a snapshot, taken at a specific moment, and we cannot assume that the problems some of our parents have faced are intrinsic to donor conception for all time. It is also important not to lose sight of the fact that our sample of parents does not include those who have no plans to tell their children about their unusual origins. We do not therefore represent their thinking and their experiences here. But we do know that this means that there will almost certainly be cohorts of young or not so young adults who discover late in life that their parent or parents are not their genetic progenitors. The consequences of the decisions taken now may still emerge in decades to come, particularly as various forms of genetic screening become more common. However, we do not know whether this discovery will, in the future, carry the significance that it appears to do in the present. Just as the experience of one's parents divorcing used to be a traumatic and isolating event for children or young adults, while now it is much more common, perhaps the discovery of non-genetic kinship will not be so devastating in future. We can, of course, only speculate on these issues.

We may be on firmer ground if we look less at the specifics of reproductive technologies and the meaning of genetics, and more at what it is that our families were trying to achieve when they opted to receive donor gametes. At one level they simply wanted to have a child or children but they all found that they had to do this against the odds for one reason or another. Having managed to achieve a conception and birth it seems that the next thing they all wanted to do was to envelop the child safely into their family, to bond with the child, and to treat the child as 'theirs' rather than as a relative stranger. They all wanted to protect the child against the consequences of being seen as different or strange and they wanted to create a strong sense of belonging which would provide a lasting ontological security for the child. In doing this, the parents and grandparents in our study had to struggle with the self-evident knowledge that each donor conceived child was 'a bit' different to other children born through so-called natural methods, but this merely drove them to greater measures to create a sense of belonging. This is the core element of the paradox of kinship, which is the title of this chapter. It is paradoxical because it seems that where genetic links may be seen as slightly attenuated, kinship links do not diminish but can strengthen to counterbalance the possible, perceived detriment. We have remarked at various stages throughout this book that kinship is complex and does not, and never has, simply followed genetic links. As part of the sometime chaos that is kinship we found that grandparents, parents and siblings can ignore difference, even forget that there are differences, or can embrace difference positively, thus making a virtue of it. How donor conception works depends very significantly on how existing networks of kinship are already working in a given family. There is not just one inevitable outcome, nor only one way of dealing with and incorporating gamete donation into family life. Families can create a sense of belonging and bonding in various ways and at times some will be more successful than others. The parents and grandparents in our study were willing to let us poke around in their family life and they revealed to us many intimate and upsetting emotions, as well as concerns about the wellbeing of their children and the need to protect them from harm. We are very grateful to them for their courage in undertaking the process. However, they did it not for our benefit alone but because they wanted other parents (and grandparents) who might be going through similar events to have the benefit of understanding the kind of experiences they had had and were still having. They hoped that their stories could begin to create a wider cultural narrative about donor conception to which new generations of parents and children could have access. In the process they hoped that donor conceived children might become less like relative strangers and more like any other family member.

Appendix I: Researching Donor Conception and Family Relationships

Our book is based on an ESRC-funded research project called 'Relative Strangers: Negotiating Non-Genetic Kinship in the Context of Assisted Conception' (RES-062-23-2810). Our primary methodology was based on in-depth interviews with 22 heterosexual parents and 22 lesbian parents of donor conceived children, and 30 additional interviews with grandparents of donor conceived children – 15 of whom had a lesbian daughter and 15 of whom had a heterosexual son or daughter. In order not to risk inadvertently conveying sensitive information to family members, we interviewed parents and grandparents from different families. Wherever possible, we interviewed couples together, but where this was impractical we interviewed people individually. We conducted 34 couple interviews and 10 individual interviews with parents (the total number of parents in the study was 78). The grandparent interviews were divided between 11 couple interviews and 19 individual interviews (in total, 41 grandparents took part). The total number of participants in the study was 119.

We did not interview children in this study because almost all of the children involved were pre-school (see below). Nor did we interview single women or include couples who were using surrogacy. Opting for donor treatment as a single woman, or for surrogacy, is a pathway likely to bring with it specific dilemmas and challenges and it deserves attention as a topic in its own right.

Recruitment

Recruitment and fieldwork took place in 2011. We recruited parents who lived in England and Wales, and who conceived using donor conception around or after 1995 when the shift towards openness started to gain momentum in the UK. We were keen to include a range of families who had conceived through different donor conception routes. We therefore avoided recruiting through clinics, and instead approached different communities and organisations, for example the Infertility Network UK/ACeBabes, The Donor Conception Network, and Fertility Friends, as well as local lesbian parent groups. Most of our recruits came through the Donor Conception Network and local Lesbian

Mums groups. We also 'snowballed' in personal and professional networks which generated some contacts.

We included grandparents whose adult children and donor conceived grandchildren lived in England or Wales, and where the children were conceived around or after 1995. Whereas there are advocacy groups organised for and by parents of donor conceived children and for lesbian mothers more specifically, there are no similar communities by or for grandparents of donor conceived children. Our only option was therefore to approach more general organisations, for example the Grandparents' Association, Saga and Grandparents Plus. This generated almost no response, and therefore we were left with the option of recruiting grandparents through parents of donor conceived children (who did not themselves take part in the study) and also through our own networks.

Collecting data

We conducted loosely structured in-depth qualitative interviews that allowed the participants to describe their lives and experiences using their own words and concepts (Kvale, 1996; Mason, 2002). The interviews contained three main elements. The first part was a conversation about a series of broad themes. These themes included how a couple came to resort to using donor conception and their experience of trying to conceive; views on sharing information about donor conception in general; decisions and processes of sharing information with the child and with the family; donor conception and everyday life (e.g. comments about family resemblances); thoughts and decisions about the donor; and approaches to information sharing more widely (i.e. within the local community, at school, with faith groups etc.). The second element comprised asking participants to map family members according to closeness on a 'closeness map' (a series of concentric circles on a paper, Smart *et al.*, 2001). This provided data in itself and the process of doing so facilitated a discussion about individual family members, disclosure and also the perceived quality of relationships in the family network. Third, we collected demographic data through a brief questionnaire that participants filled in themselves. When deemed helpful, we also added a fourth element to the interview, which was that we presented the interviewees with a short story about a parent or grandparent of a donor conceived child, who faced an ethical dilemma of information sharing. We asked the interviewee to offer their advice to the parent/grandparent in the story.

The interviews lasted between one and two hours. We recorded the interviews digitally and they were thereafter transcribed verbatim and anonymised.

Sample composition

Among the 74 families we interviewed, 54 couples had conceived using sperm donation, 16 egg donation, 3 embryo donation and 1 both sperm and embryo donation (this family had a first child through sperm donation and were expecting a second through embryo donation). Many couples had more than one donor conceived child, and the total number of donor conceived children in the families in the study was 111 (including five pregnancies where the children were due to be born in 2011). Usually, when couples had donor conceived siblings they had been conceived using the same type of gamete donation (either donor egg or sperm for example), but as indicated above, in one interview a couple had their first-born by sperm donation and the second by embryo donation. Table A1 (below) indicates the split between the number of children born through sperm, egg and embryo donation in the families in the study.

Table A1 indicates that the number of sperm donation cases is the main form of gamete donation in our study. Sperm donation is a far more common treatment option in the UK compared with egg donation and embryo donation (Human Fertilisation and Embryology Authority, 2013d). We also had a focus in the study on lesbian couples and their families, in which almost all spoke of sperm donation only. Looking specifically at the cases of heterosexual donation (comprising 22 parent interviews and 15 grandparent interviews), there were 18 cases of sperm donation, 16 of egg donation and 3 of embryo donation.

The study also included a diverse range of different donor conception pathways, including licensed UK clinics, clinics abroad, self-arranged sperm donation and Internet company providers of donor sperm, as highlighted by Table A2.

Table A2 shows that in 77 per cent of cases children were conceived through clinical reproductive health treatment, and in 18 per cent of cases self-arranged practices were used. Fewer than 3 per cent of the families had children conceived both through clinical and self-arranged donor conception, and fewer than 3 per cent (2 cases) had used an Internet company provider.

Looking at the cases of lesbian donation in our data (including 22 interviews with parents and the 15 with grandparents), the couples had conceived using either clinical conception (20), self-arranged conception (13), both clinical and self-arranged (2) or conception through an Internet company provider (2), indicating that the group of lesbian parents in this study tended to use

Table A1 Number of children conceived in the study by gamete donation type (total number of children in the families in the study $N = 111$)

Type of gamete	Number of children	Percentage
Sperm donation	84	76
Egg donation	23	21
Embryo donation	4	< 4
Total	111	100

Table A2 Frequency of route to conception (total number of cases $N = 74$)

Conception route	Number	Percentage
Clinical conception	57	77
(Of whom conceived in CBRC)[1]	(6)	
Self-arranged conception	13	18
Clinical and self-arranged	2	< 3
Internet company provider	2	< 3
Total	74	100

diverse donor conception practices. By contrast, the cases of heterosexual donation were far more homogenous as all couples had taken the clinic route (either in the UK or abroad).

Age and location

The youngest parent in the study was 25 years old at the time of the interview (a lesbian mother born in 1986) and the oldest family member (a great-grandmother of an embryo donor child) was 89 years old, born in 1922. The oldest donor conceived child or grandchild referred to was born in 1987, and the youngest were born, or due to be born, in 2011. Table A3 outlines the age spread in the different groups in our sample.

Table A3 indicates that youngest parent was born in 1986 compared to the oldest parent who was born in 1956. The median parent in the study was born in 1970 and so was at the time of the interview 41 years of age. The median donor conceived child in the study was born in 2008, and so was three years old at the time of the interview in 2011.

Table A3 Birth year of participants and donor conceived children in families interviewed ($N = 229$)

Generation groups	Oldest birth year	Youngest birth year	Median birth year	Number of participants and donor conceived children in their families
Grandparents	1922	1953	1943	41
Parents	1956	1986	1970	78
Children	1987	2011	2008	111
Total				229

The interviewees lived in both rural and urban locations in England and Wales. The participants who lived in urban locations were particularly clustered in the Greater London area (16) and in Manchester (11). In four cases, grandparents lived outside England and Wales, and were to be found in Scotland, Spain, Belgium and the US (but their children and grandchildren resided in the UK).

Gender, ethnicity, religion and socio-economic status

More women than men took part in our study and 90 of the 119 participants were women. This gender difference was in part explained by our focus on lesbian couples and in part by the fact that women predominantly came forward for individual interviews in both the parent and grandparent samples. This difference was particularly stark in the grandparent interviews where a much higher proportion of the interviewees (70 per cent of the total of 41 grandparents) were women.

Ninety-nine (or 83 per cent) of the men and women who took part identified as white British (including Scottish, Welsh and English identities) (see Table A4). In addition, 13 individuals identified as white European, American or Australian. Four individuals identified as mixed British and three as Asian.

In terms of religion, over half of our interviewees (53 per cent) identified as atheist or agnostic. But there was also a substantial group of people of different Christian faiths in the study (40 per cent). A limited proportion identified as Jewish (5 per cent), while no one of Muslim faith came forward to be interviewed. Two per cent chose not to reveal their faith.

Following Graham (2007: 55), we used education as a measure of class linking parental social class and the respondents' own class. Among all 119 participants, 30 per cent (36 individuals) had as their highest qualification GCESs, A-levels or further education diplomas, most of which had been

Table A4 Ethnic identity of participants (total number of participants $N = 119$)

Ethnicity	Number	Percent
White British identities (including Scottish, Welsh, English)	99	83
White European, American or Australian identities	13	11
Mixed British identities (Chinese/British (1), British/Asian (1), British/ European (2))	4	3
Asian identities (Chinese (1), Indian (1), Pakistani (1))	3	< 3
Total	119	100

Table A5 Parent participants' highest level of qualification (total number of parents $N = 78$)

Highest level of education	Number	Percent
GSCEs, A-level, or further education qualification	16	21
Higher education qualification	61	78
Unassigned	1	1
Total	78	100

acquired by the age of 18. In contrast, over two-thirds (or 68 per cent) had a higher education qualification. Looking at the parent group specifically, their qualification outline is highlighted in Table A5.

Table A5 suggests that among our parent participants, 21 per cent had left full-time education by the age of 18 while 78 per cent had gone on to higher education. Compared with the general population of women giving birth in Britain (Dex and Joshi, 2004), this gives a broad indication that the parent group we interviewed were disproportionately middle class, which was also true for the sample more generally.

Sample profile: Some issues

It is important to appreciate the significance for our study of the fact that the Donor Conception Network became such a crucial gateway for recruiting participants because the majority of the heterosexual parents were recruited in this way. The Donor Conception Network is an advocacy group for openness in the context of donor conception. We are therefore more likely to have recruited couples who are committed to openness than those who have decided to keep the donor conception secret. We also – for obvious reasons – only recruited grandparents who knew all about the donor conception, but in addition it was more likely that they had a good relationship with their adult children and were relatively happy with the arrangements they had made to have children. It was unlikely that a parent whose own parents deeply disagreed with the practice of donor conception would volunteer them for the study, and it was equally unlikely that such grandparents would agree to take part. Due to our recruitment process, the study is more likely to highlight how openness impacts on family networks, rather than secrecy.

The data is also likely to be shaped by the specificities of the sample. Our study mainly reflects experiences of conception using donor sperm and donor eggs, but we were far less able to recruit family members of children conceived using embryo donation. The sample profile outlined above also suggests that the study mainly explored the experiences of donor conception among white British, atheist, agnostic or Church of England middle-class families. The over-representation of women in the study also suggests that we were more able to tap into women's experiences of donor conception and family life than men's. With a different sample composition, the data might also have looked different.

Ethical considerations

Donor conception can give rise to secrets in family networks and so as part of designing the study it was necessary to resolve the ethical dilemmas related to doing research about issues that potentially raise sensitivities in families. A central dilemma was avoiding inadvertent exposure of family secrets in family networks because this might greatly affect family dynamics and relationships in irreversible ways (Smart, 2011). To conduct the study ethically, it was therefore particularly important that we designed a research process where we could safeguard the anonymity and confidentiality of all participants (Social Research Association, 2003). We decided that this would only be fully possible if we interviewed parents and grandparents from different families. This meant that we were not able to bring together the voices from parents and grandparents from the same family who reflect on the same relationship from different perspectives. Instead we have a large number of families represented in the study, highlighted through the perspective of either parents or grandparents. To protect the participants, all names, places and identifying details have been anonymised.

Appendix II: Index of Participants

Key

Case Number	Two Names (+ages)	Couple interview with both partners
Case Number	One Name (+partner/ages)	Individual interview, partner not present
Case Number	One Name only (+age)	Individual interview, separated or divorced

100s: Lesbian parents

Case number	Name(s) and age	Brief outline
101	Amy (34) and Jessica (38)	Twins through donor sperm and IVF, UK clinic. Identity release donor.
102	Stacey (36)	One daughter through self-arranged conception. Donor known but uninvolved.
103	Julia (34) and Molly (45)	One son and one daughter through clinical sperm donor conception, UK. Identity release donor. Both children same donor. Same birth mother.
104	Vanessa (45)	Twins through donor sperm and IVF, UK clinic. Same donor. Donor known; family member. Donor uninvolved in parenting.
105	Amber (32) and Heather (27)	One son through clinical sperm donor conception, UK clinic. Identity release donor.
106	Danielle (44) (partner Christina)	One son through clinical sperm donor conception UK, identity release donor. Expecting a sibling through embryo donation, conceived in clinic abroad. Donors for sibling anonymous. Same birth mother.
107	Angela (34) and Samantha (41)	One son through self-arranged conception. Donor known as Dad.

(Continued)

Case number	Name(s) and age	Brief outline
108	Laura (42) and Natalie (34)	One son through self-arranged conception. Known donor, but he is uninvolved in the family.
109	Alison (40) and Beth (36)	One son through clinical sperm donation, UK. Expecting a second child, also through UK licensed clinic. Both children same donor. Different birth mothers.
110	Bridget (25) and Lori (42)	One son through self-arranged conception, and expecting a sibling. Donor known but uninvolved as a parent. Same birth mother.
111	Dawn (49) and Linda (31)	One son through self-arranged conception Known donor, but he is uninvolved in the family.
112	Tabetha (40) and Tina (44)	One son through clinical sperm donation, UK. Identity release donor.
113	Meredith (36) and Priscilla (36)	Two sons through clinical sperm donation, UK. Donor anonymous. Both children same donor. Same birth mother.
114	Gemma (41) and Sasha (43)	Two daughters, clinical sperm donation, UK. First child anonymous donor, second child identity release donor. Different donor. Same birth mother.
115	Sheryl (38)	One daughter, self-arranged donor insemination. Donor known but uninvolved.
116	Claudia (40) and Nina (30)	Expecting a child, self-arranged donor insemination. Donor known but uninvolved.
117	Malinda (38) and Robyn (35)	One daughter through self-arranged donor insemination. Donor known but uninvolved in the family. Donor associated with the wider family.
118	Michelle (34) and Sharon (30)	One daughter through Internet company provider of donor sperm. Couple unsure if donor is anonymous or can be identified.

119	Alexandra (38) and Karen (39)	One daughter and one son through donor sperm and IVF, UK clinic. Identity release donor, same donor both children. Different birth mothers.
120	Susan (53)	Three children across two relationships. One son and one daughter conceived through self-arranged sperm donation. Anonymous donors, different for the two children. Different birth mothers. Third child (son) through clinical donor insemination, UK clinic. Donor identity release. Non-birth mother of the third son.
121	Jenny (44) and Miranda (49)	One daughter through clinical sperm donation. Donor initially anonymous, but has opted for identity release.
122	Lauren (50) and Olivia (42)	Two sons through sperm donation in a UK clinic. Donor known but uninvolved in parenting.

200s: Heterosexual couples

Case number	Name(s)	Brief outline
201	Cathryn (51) and Daniel (51)	Two daughters through egg donation, UK clinic. Different donors for the two children. First donor anonymous, second identity release.
202	Zoe (43) and Matthew (47)	Three sons through donor insemination, UK clinic. Same donor all children. Donor anonymous.
203	Delia (39) and James (40)	One daughter through donor sperm, UK clinic. Identity release donor.
204	Fiona (49) and Brian (39)	One daughter through egg donation, UK clinic. Donor anonymous.
205	Martha (55) and Nicholas (54)	One son through egg donation, UK. Donor anonymous.
206	Lea (37) and Joshua (50)	One daughter through donor sperm and IVF, UK. Donor identity release.

(Continued)

Case number	Name(s)	Brief outline
207	Christine (39) and Jared (43)	Two sons through clinical donor insemination, UK. Same donor both children. Donor anonymous.
208	Carrie (44) (partner Paul)	One son and one daughter through sperm donation, UK clinic. Same donor both children. Donor anonymous.
209	Erica (41) and Kevin (49)	One son and one daughter through sperm donation, UK clinic. Same donor both children. Identity release donor.
210	Jennifer (36) and Robert (37)	Two daughters through donor insemination, UK clinic. Same donor both children. Identity release donor.
211	Brenda (46) and Jeremy (47)	Twins egg donation. Clinic abroad, donor anonymous.
212	Victoria (38) (partner Jeffrey)	One son and one daughter through donor insemination, UK clinic. Imported sperm from abroad. Same donor both children. Identity release donor.
213	Monica (37) and Trevor (36)	One daughter through sperm donation, UK clinic. Identity release donor.
214	Stephanie (41) and Clive (40)	One son through egg donation, expecting a sibling through egg donation. UK clinic. Same donor both children. Donor anonymous.
215	Elaine (48) and Timothy (54)	One daughter through donor insemination, UK clinic. Donor anonymous.
216	Melissa (38) and David (38)	One son through egg donation, UK clinic. Donor known, but uninvolved in parenting.
217	Erin (44) (partner Adam)	One daughter through egg donation, UK clinic. Identity release donor.
218	Holly (49) and Patrick (45)	One son through egg donation, UK clinic. Donor known, but uninvolved in parenting.
219	Cathleen (54)	Two sons and one daughter through sperm donation, UK clinic. Different donors, all donors anonymous.

220	Cara (51) (partner Angus)	One daughter through sperm donation, UK clinic. Donor anonymous.
221	Elizabeth (37) and Adrian (36)	One son through sperm donation, UK clinic. Identity release donor.
222	Abigail (48) and Jonathan (44)	One son through egg donation, UK clinic. Donor known, uninvolved in parenting.

300s: Grandparents through lesbian donation

Case number	Name(s)	Brief outline
301	Denise (59) and Donald (61)	Genetic grandparents of one grandchild through clinical sperm donor conception, UK. Non-genetic grandparents of second grandchild through self-arranged donor insemination.
302	Nancy (68) (partner Joseph)	Non-genetic grandmother of two children through clinical sperm donor conception. UK clinic.
303	Theresa (67)	Genetic grandmother of two grandchildren through clinical sperm donor conception, UK.
304	Judith (69)	Genetic grandmother of one child through donor conception. Believed daughter conceived through private arrangement with donor.
305	Meg (73)	Two genetic grandchildren and one non-genetic grandchild through clinical sperm donor conception, UK.
306	Anita (58) and Tony (61)	Non-genetic grandparents of child conceived using self-arranged sperm donation. Donor known but uninvolved in parenting.
307	Margaret (69)	Non-genetic grandchild through clinical donor insemination, UK.
308	Louisa (65)	Genetic grandmother of a grandchild conceived using clinical sperm donation, UK.

(Continued)

Case number	Name(s)	Brief outline
309	Irene (76)	One genetic grandchild and one non-genetic grandchild. Children conceived in self-arranged sperm donation. Donor uninvolved in parenting. Same donor.
310	Veronica (72) and Howard (82)	Veronica the genetic grandparent of a child conceived using self-arranged sperm donation. Howard her husband. Donor involved as a parent.
311	Valerie (62) and Alan (62)	Valarie the genetic grandparent of a child conceived using sperm donation provided by Internet company. Alan her husband.
312	Maureen (64)	One genetic grandchild through clinical sperm donation, UK.
313	Vivian (68) and Keith (77)	One genetic grandchild through clinical sperm donation and IVF, UK.
314	Betty (67) and Richard (69)	One non-genetic grandchild through clinical sperm donation, UK.
315	Annette (65)	One non-genetic grandchild through self-arranged sperm donation. Donor uninvolved in parenting.

400s: Grandparents through heterosexual donation

Case number	Name(s)	Brief outline
401	Hannah (68)	Non-genetic grandchild conceived using egg donation. Egg donor part of family, uninvolved in parenting.
402	Leonard (69)	Non-genetic grandchild conceived using egg donation. Donor known, part of wider family. Donor uninvolved in parenting.
403	Alice (87)	Four non-genetic grandchildren by egg donation, clinic US. Same donor.
404	Joyce (63) and Kenneth (63)	Joyce the genetic grandmother of a child conceived using clinical sperm donation, UK. Kenneth her husband.

405	Wendy (67)	Genetic grandmother of a child conceived using clinical sperm donation, UK.
406	Barbara (68) and William (67)	The non-genetic grandparents of a grandchild by sperm donation, UK clinic.
407	Sheila (74) and Philip (79)	Non-genetic grandparents of a child conceived using embryo donation, clinic abroad.
408	Joanne (85)	Genetic grandmother of a child conceived using egg donation, clinic abroad.
409	Shirley (79)	Non-genetic grandmother of a child conceived using egg donation, UK clinic.
410	Lisa (66) and Roger (67)	Genetic grandparents of two grandchildren conceived using sperm donation, UK clinic.
411	Sally (64)	Non-genetic grandmother of a child conceived using embryo donation, UK clinic.
412	Phyllis (89)	Non-genetic great-grandmother of a child conceived using embryo donation, UK clinic.
413	Frances (72)	Non-genetic grandmother of twins conceived using egg donation, UK clinic.
414	Jacqueline (74)	Non-genetic grandmother of a child conceived using egg donation, clinic abroad. Known donor, but involved.
415	Sarah (68) and Norman (71)	Genetic grandparents of a child conceived using sperm donation, UK clinic.

Appendix III: Glossary of terms

Abbreviation	Full title	Explanation
Egg donation		The process whereby a woman provides one or several eggs for assisted reproduction or research. Eggs fertilised in vitro and then implanted into recipient.
Embryo donation		The donation of embryos for assisted reproduction or research. Embryos formed in vitro. Implanted into the recipient.
HFE Act	Human Fertilisation and Embryology Act	The act of the parliament of the UK regulating assisted conception practices and research. First Act 1990, revised in 2008.
HFEA	Human Fertilisation and Embryology Authority	The UK's independent regulator overseeing the use of gametes and embryos in fertility treatment and research. Also licenses fertility clinics carrying out assisted conception procedures and human embryo research.[1]
ICSI	Intra-Cytoplasmic Sperm Injection	Injection of a single sperm into an egg in vitro in order to fertilise it.
IVF	In vitro fertilisation	When an egg is fertilised by sperm outside the body, in vitro.
IUI	Intrauterine insemination	The process of inserting sperm directly into the uterus (womb) at the time of ovulation.
Sperm donation		The process whereby a man provides sperm for third party conception or research. Can either take place in a reproductive health care centre or be self-arranged.
Gamete		A cell that fuses with another cell during fertilisation.

Notes

Introduction

1. Human Fertilisation and Embryology Authority 2013b.

1 Proper Families? Cultural Expectations and Donor Conception

1. For example, the notorious Section 28 of the 1988 Local Government Act forbade local authorities from intentionally promoting homosexuality or publishing material with the intention of promoting homosexuality, or from promoting the teaching in any maintained school of the acceptability of homosexuality as a pretended family relationship. This was only repealed in England and Wales in 2003.
2. The correct citation for this case is *ML & AR v RW & SW [2011] EWHC 2455 (Fam)*, with a subsequent judgment to be found at *P & L (Minors) [2011] EWHC 3431*. The parties to the conflict are anonymous but in order to facilitate the story we have given fictitious names to the people involved.
3. A really surprising instance of this became public knowledge when Sir Paul Nurse, President of the Royal Society and Nobel prize–winning geneticist, discovered in later life that his sister was in fact his mother. Sir Paul was born in 1948, long after the Adoption Act was implemented, and yet it is clear that this kind of practice still went on in families, perhaps especially during and immediately after the war.

2 Uncharted Territories: Donor Conception in Personal Life

1. The situation with egg donors could be different, especially where donors were family members. But where they were not, a suitable 'distance' was required (see Chapter 7).

5 Opening Up: Disclosure, Information and Family Relationships

1. The DCN was formed in the early 1990s by a handful of parents of donor conceived children. It is an advocate group for disclosure in the field of donor conception which has been highly influential in promoting openness in the UK. It has grown significantly in size and influence since, and, in 2013 counted 1600 families as members. The DCN works, among other things, to educate parents about the importance of openness and also to support and guide parents in sharing information openly.

6 Relating to Donors: Strangers, Boundaries and Tantalising Knowledge

1. Some had conceived in donation programmes where the donor would always remain anonymous; others had donors whose identities could be released when the child reached adulthood.

8 Relative Strangers and the Paradoxes of Genetic Kinship

1. Carsten (2004), Edwards (2000), Franklin (2003), Howell (2003), Inhorn (2007), Konrad (2005), Mason (2008) and Nahman (2013).

Appendix I: Researching Donor Conception and Family Relationships

1. The six couples who conceived through CBRB had received treatment in Spain (1), the Czech Republic (2), the US (2) and Canada (1).

Appendix III: Glossary of terms

1. HFEA 2013 http://www.hfea.gov.uk/index.html

Bibliography

Adair, R. (1996) *Courtship, Illegitimacy and Marriage in Early Modern England*, Manchester: Manchester University Press.

Adie, K. (2005) *Nobody's Child: Who are You When You Don't Know Your Past?* London: Hodder & Stoughton.

Allan, G. and Crow, G. (2001) *Families, Households and Society*, Basingstoke: Palgrave.

Almack, K. (2007) 'Out and about: Negotiating the layers of being out in the process of disclosure of lesbian parenthood', *Sociological Research Online*, 12(1).

Anderson, B. (2006; orig 1983) *Imagined Communities*, London: Verso.

Appleby, J., Blake, L. and Freeman, T. (2012) 'Is disclosure in the best interest of children conceived by donation?' in M. Richards, G. Pennings and J. Appleby (eds) *Reproductive Donation: Practice, Policy and Bioethics*, pp. 231–249, Cambridge: Cambridge University Press.

Becker, G. (2000) *The Elusive Embryo: How Women and Men Approach New Reproductive Technologies*, Berkeley, Los Angeles, London: University of California Press.

Becker, G., Butler, A. and Nachtigall, R. D. (2005) 'Resemblance talk: A challenge for parents whose children were conceived with donor gametes in the US', *Social Science and Medicine*, 61:1300–1309.

Bengtson, V., Biblarz, T. J. and Roberts, R. E. L. (2002) *How Families Still Matter: A Longitudinal Study of Youth in Two Generations*, Cambridge: Cambridge University Press.

Bloklan, T. (2005) 'Memory Magic: How a working-class neighbourhood became an imagined community and class started to matter when it lost its base', in Devine, F. *et al.* (eds) *Rethinking Class*, pp. 123–139, Basingstoke: Palgrave Macmillan.

Blyth, E., Frith, L., Jones, C. and Speirs, J. M. (2009) 'The role of birth certificates in relation to access to biographical and genetic history in donor conception', *International Journal of Children's Rights*, 17(2): 207–233.

Brannen, J., Moss, P. and Mooney, A. (2004) *Working and Caring over the Twentieth Century*, Basingstoke: Palgrave Macmillan.

Carey, N. (2012) *The Epigenics Revolution*, London: Faber & Faber.

Carsten, J. (2001) 'Substantivism, antisubstantivism and anti-antisubstantivism', in S. Franklin and S. McKinnon (eds) *Relative Values: Reconfiguring Kinship Studies*, pp. 29–53, Durham: Duke University Press.

Carsten, J. (2004) *After Kinship*, Cambridge: Cambridge University Press.

Cowden, M. (2012) 'No harm, no foul': A child's right to know their genetic parents', *International Journal of Law, Policy and the Family*, 26(1): 102–126.

Culley, L. and Hudson, N. (2006) 'Disrupted reproduction and deviant bodies: Pronatalism and British South Asian communities', *International Journal of Diversity Organisations, Communities and Nations*, 5: 117–126.

Culley, L., Hudson, N., Rapport, F., Blyth, W., Norton, E. and Pacey, A. A. (2011) 'Crossing borders for fertility treatment: Motivations, destinations and outcomes of UK fertility travellers', *Human Reproduction*, 26(9): 2373–2381.

Daniels, K. R., Lewis, G. M., and Gillett, W. R. (1995) 'Telling donor insemination offspring about their conception: The nature of couples' decision making', *Social Science and Medicine*, 40(9): 1213–1220.

Daniels, K. R., Grace, V. M. and Gillett, W. R. (2011) 'Factors associated with parents' decisions to tell their adult offspring about the offspring's donor conception', *Human Reproduction*, 26(10): 2783–2790.

Daniels, K. and Haimes, E. (eds) (1998) *Donor Insemination: International Social Science Perspectives*, Cambridge: Cambridge University Press.

Dawkins, R. (1976) *The Selfish Gene*, Oxford: Oxford University Press.

Degnen, C. (2009) 'Eating genes and raising people', in Edwards, J. and Salazar, C. (eds) *European Kinship in the Age of Biotechnology*, pp. 45–63, Oxford: Berghahn Books.

Dex, S. and Joshi, H. (2004) *Millennium Cohort Study First Survey: The User's Guide to Initial Findings*, Centre for Longitudinal Studies, Bedford Group for Lifecourse and Statistical Studies, Institute of Education, London: University of London.

Donovan, C. (2000) 'Who needs a father? Negotiating biological fatherhood in British lesbian families using self-insemination', *Sexualities*, 3(2): 149–164.

Edwards, J. (2000) *Born and Bred: Idioms of Kinship and New Reproductive Technologies in England*, Oxford: Oxford University Press.

Edwards, J. (forthcoming) 'Understanding kinship and relatedness through assisted conception', in T. Freeman, S. Graham, F. Ebtehaj, and M. Richards (eds) *Relatedness in Assisted Reproduction: Families, Origins and Identities*, Cambridge: Cambridge University Press.

Edwards, J. and Salazar, C. (eds) (2009) *European Kinship in the Age of Biotechnology*, Oxford: Berghahn Books.

Fenton, R. A. (2006) 'Catholic doctrine versus women's rights: The new Italian law on assisted reproduction', *Medical Law Review*, 14 (Spring): 73–107.

Finch, J. (1989) *Family Obligations and Social Change*, Cambridge: Polity.

Finch, J. and Mason, J. (1993) *Negotiating Family Responsibilities*, London: Tavistock/Routledge.

Franklin, S. (1997) *Embodied Progress*, London: Routledge.

Franklin, S. (2003) 'Rethinking nature-culture: Anthropology and the new genetics', *Anthropological Theory*, 3(1):65–85.

Gillis, J. (1996) *A World of Their Own Making*, Boston, Massachusetts: Harvard University Press.

Goffman, E. (1990, orig. 1959) *The Presentation of Self in Everyday Life*, Harmondsworth: Penguin.

Gottlieb, C., Lalos, O. and Lindblad, F. (2000) 'Legislated right for donor-insemination children to know their genetic origin: A study of parental thinking', *Human Reproduction*, 15(9): 2052–2056.

Grace, V. and Daniels, K. R. (2007) 'The (ir)relevance of genetics: Engendering parallel worlds of procreation and reproduction', *Sociology of Health & Illness*, 29(5): 692–710.

Grace, V., Daniels, K.R., Gillett, W. (2008) 'The donor, the father, and the imaginary constitution of the family: Parents' constructions in the case of donor insemination', *Social Science and Medicine*, 66(2): 301–314.

Graham, H. (2007) *Unequal Lives: Health and Socio-economic Inequalities*, Maidenhead: Open University Press.

Guichon, J. R., Mitchell, I. and Giroux, M. (eds) (2012) *The Right to Know one's Origins: Assisted Human Reproduction and the Best Interests of Children*, Brussels: Academic and Scientific Publishers.

Haimes, E. (1988) 'Secrecy: What can artificial reproduction learn from adoption?' *International Journal of Law, Policy and the Family*, 2(1): 46–61.

Haimes, E. (1992) 'Gamete donation and the social management of genetic origins', pp. 119–147 in M. Stacey (ed) *Changing Human Reproduction: Social Science Perspectives*, London: Sage.

Haraway, D. (1997) *Modest_Witness@Second_Millennium. FemaleMan©_Meets_OncoMouse™*, London: Routledge.

Howell, S. (2001) 'Self-conscious kinship: Some contested values in Norwegian transnational adoption', in S. Franklin and S. McKinnon (eds) *Relative Values: Reconfiguring Kinship Studies*, pp. 203–223 Durham and London: Duke University Press.

Howell, S. (2003) 'Kinning: The creation of life trajectories in transnational adoptive families, *Journal of the Royal Anthropological Institute*, 9:465–484.

Human Fertilisation and Embryology Authority (2013a) 'Long-term trends data – patients treated', Accessed at <http://www.hfea.gov.uk/2585.html> 30 May 2013.

Human Fertilisation and Embryology Authority (2013b) 'Sperm websites', Accessed at <http://www.hfea.gov.uk/1369.html> 30 May 2013.

Human Fertilisation and Embryology Authority (2013c) 'Family limit for donated sperm and eggs', Accessed at <http://www.hfea.gov.uk/6192.html> 31 January 2013.

HFEA (2013d) 'Long term data - birth rates', Accessed at <http://www.hfea.gov.uk/2588.html> 30 May 2013.

Inhorn, M. C. (2007) 'Reproductive disruptions and assisted reproductive technologies in the Muslim world', in Marcia Inhorn (ed) *Reproductive Disruptions*, Oxford: Berghahn Books.

Inness, J. (1992) *Privacy, Intimacy and Isolation*, Oxford: Oxford University Press.

Isaksson, S., Skoog Svanberg, A., Sydsjo, G., Thurin-Kjellberg, A., Karlström, P-O., Solensten, N-G. and Lampic, C. (2011) 'Two decades after legislation on identifiable donors in Sweden: Are recipient couples ready to be open about using gamete donation?' *Human Reproduction*, 26(4): 853–860.

Jones, C. and Hackett, S. (2012) 'Redefining family relationships following adoption: Adoptive parents' perspectives on the changing nature of kinship between adoptees and birth relatives', *British Journal of Social Work*, 42: 283–299.

Jones, S. (1993) *The Language of the Genes*, London: Flamingo.

Jones, S. (1996) *In the Blood: God, Genes and Destiny*, London: Flamingo.

Keating, J. (2009) *A Child for Keeps: The History of Adoption in England, 1918–45*, Basingstoke: Palgrave Macmillan.

Kirkman, M. (2003) 'Parents' contributions to the narrative identity of offspring of donor-assisted conception', *Social Science & Medicine* 57(11): 2229–2242.

Kirkman, M. (2005) 'Going home and forgetting about it: Donor insemination and the secrecy debate', in H. G. Jones and M. Kirkman (eds) *Sperm Wars: The Rights and Wrongs of Reproduction*, pp. 153–169, Sydney: Australian Broadcasting Cooperation.

Konrad, M. (2005) *Nameless Relations*, Oxford: Berghahn Books.

Kvale, S. (1996) *Inter Views*, London: Sage.

Lalos, A., Gottlieb, C. and Lalos, O. (2007) 'Legislated right for donor-insemination children to know their genetic origin: A study of parental thinking', *Human Reproduction*, 22(6): 1759–1768.

Landau, R. and Weissenberg, R. (2010) 'Disclosure of donor conception in single-mother families: Views and concerns', *Human Reproduction*, 25(4): 942–948.

Laruelle, C., Place, I., Demeestere, I., Englert, Y. and Delbaere, A. (2011) 'Anonymity and secrecy options of recipient couples and donors, and ethnic origin influence in three types of oocyte donation', *Human Reproduction*, 26(2): 382–390.

Laslett, P. (2000, orig 1965) *The World we have Lost – Further Explained*, London: Routledge.

Lawler, S. (2008) *Identity*, Cambridge: Polity.

Lewis, J. (2001) *The End of Marriage?* Cheltenham: Edward Elgar.

Lewis, J. (2004) 'Adoption: The nature of policy shifts in England and Wales, 1972–2002', *International Journal of Law, Policy and the Family* (18): 235–255.

Lorbach, C. (2003) *Experiences of Donor Conception*, London: Jessica Kingsley Publishers.

MacCallum, F. (2009) 'Embryo donation parents' attitudes towards donors: Comparison with adoption', *Human Reproduction*, 24(3): 517–523.

Mamo, L. (2007) *Queering Reproduction: Achieving Pregnancy in the Age of Technoscience*, Durham: Duke University Press.

Marre, D. and Bestard, J. (2009) 'The family body: Persons, bodies and resemblance', in J. Edwards and C. Salazar (eds) *European Kinship in the Age of Biotechnology*, Fertility, Reproduction and Sexuality series, pp. 64–78. Oxford: Berghahn Books.

Marshall, J. (2012) 'Concealed births, adoption and human rights law: Being wary of seeking to open windows into people's souls', *The Cambridge Law Journal*, 71(2): 325–354.

Martin, E. (2001) *The Woman in the Body*, Boston: Beacon Press.

Mason, J. (2002) *Qualitative Researching*, 2nd edn., London: Sage.

Mason, J. (2008) 'Tangible affinities and the real life fascination of kinship', *Sociology*, 42(1): 29–45.

Mason, J., May, V. and Clarke, L. (2007) 'Ambivalence and the paradoxes of grandparenting', *The Sociological Review*, 55(4): 687–706.

May, V. (2013) *Connecting Self to Society*, Basingstoke: Palgrave Macmillan.

McRae, S. (2004) *Changing Britain: Family and Household in the 1990s*, Oxford: Oxford University Press.

Midgley, M. (2010) *The Solitary Self: Darwin and the Selfish Gene*, Durham: Acumen Publishing Ltd.

Morgan, D. (1996) *Family Connections: An Introduction to Family Studies*, Cambridge: Polity Press.

Morgan, D. (2011) *Rethinking Family Practices*, Basingstoke: Palgrave Macmillan.

Morgan, P. (1995) *Farewell to the Family?*, London: Institute of Economic Affairs, Choice in Welfare Series No 21.

Morgan, P. (2000) *Marriage-Lite: The Rise of Cohabitation and its Consequences*, London: Institute for the Study of Civil Society.

Murray, C. and Golombok, S. (2003) 'To tell or not to tell: The decision-making process of egg-donation parents', *Human Fertility*, 6(2):89–95.

Nahman, M.R. (2013) *Extractions: An Ethnography of Reproductive Tourism*, Palgrave Macmillan: Basingstoke Nippert-Eng, C. (2010) *Islands of Privacy*, Chicago: The University of Chicago.

Nordqvist, P. (2010) ' "Out of sight, out of mind": Family resemblances in lesbian donor conception', *Sociology*, 44(6): 1128–1144.

Nordqvist, P. (2011a) 'Choreographies of sperm donations: Dilemmas of intimacy in lesbian couple donor conception', *Social Science and Medicine*, 73(11): 1661–1668.

Nordqvist, P. (2011b) 'Dealing with sperm: Comparing lesbians' clinical and non-clinical donor conception processes', *Sociology of Health and Illness*, 33: 114–129.

Nordqvist, P. (2012a) 'Origins and originators: Lesbian couples negotiating parental identities and sperm donor conception', *Culture, Health and Sexuality*, 14(3): 297–311.

Nordqvist, P. (2012b) ' "I don't want us to stand out more than we already do": Complexities and negotiations in lesbian couples' accounts of becoming a family through donor conception', *Sexualities*, 15(5–6): 644–661.

Nordqvist, P. and Smart, C. (forthcoming) 'Relational lives, relational selves: Assisted conception and intergenerational relationships', in T. Freeman, S. Graham, F. Ebtehaj, and M. Richards (eds) *Relatedness in Assisted Reproduction: Families, Origins and Identities*, Cambridge: Cambridge University Press.

Nuffield Council on Bioethics (2013) *Donor Conception: Ethical Aspects of Information Sharing*, London: Nuffield Council on Bioethics.

Ponse, B. (1976) 'Secrecy in the lesbian world', *Journal of Contemporary Ethnography*, 5(3): 313–338.

Readings, J., Blake, L., Casey, P., Vasanti, J. and Golombok, S. (2011) 'Secrecy, disclosure and everything in-between: Decisions of parents of children conceived by donor insemination, egg donation and surrogacy', *Reproductive BioMedicine Online*, 22(5): 485–495.

Richards, J. (2008) *'The innocent have nothing to hide': exploring the notion and practice of 'privacy' in everyday life*, unpublished master's thesis, University of Manchester.

Richards, M. (2006) 'Genes, genealogies and paternity: making babies in the twenty-first century', in J. R. Spencer and A. du Bois-Pedain (eds) *Freedom and Responsibility in Reproductive Choice*, pp. 53–73, Oxford: Hart Publishing.

Richards, M., Pennings, G. and Appleby, J. (eds) (2012) *Reproductive Donation: Practice, Policy and Bioethics*, Cambridge: Cambridge University Press.

Rights of Women (1984) *Lesbian Mothers on Trial. A Report On Lesbian Mothers and Child Custody*, London: Rights of Women.

Rose, J. (2012) 'Identity harm: Lessons from adoption for donor conception' in Guichon, J. R., Mitchell, I. and Giroux, M. (eds) *The Right to Know one's Origins: Assisted Human Reproduction and the Best Interests of Children*, pp. 106–120, Brussels: Academic and Scientific Publishers.

Rose, H. and Rose, S. (2012) *Genes, Cells and Brains: The Promethean Promises of the New Biology*, London: Verso.

Rose, S. (1997) *Lifelines: Life beyond the Gene*, Oxford: Oxford University Press.

Rose, S., Lewontin, R. C. and Kamin, L. J. (1984) *Not in Our Genes: Biology, Ideology and Human Nature*, Harmondsworth: Pelican Books.

Sales, S. (2012) *Adoption, Family and the Paradox of Origins. A Foucauldian History*, Basingstoke: Palgrave Macmillan.

Shenfield, F., de Mouzon, J., Pennings, G., Ferraretti, A. P., Nyboe Andersen, A., de Wert, G., Goossens, V., The ESHRE Taskforce on Cross Border Reproductive Care (2010) 'Cross border reproductive care in six European Countries', *Human Reproduction*, 25(6): 1361–1368.

Smart, C. (1987) ' "There is of course the distinction dictated by nature": Law and the problem of paternity', in Michelle Stanworth (ed) *Reproductive Technologies*, pp. 98–117, Cambridge: Polity.

Smart, C. (2007) *Personal Life: New Directions in Sociological Thinking*, Cambridge: Polity.

Smart, C. (2011) 'Families, secrets and memories', *Sociology*, 45: 539.

Smart, C. and Neale, B. (1999) *Family Fragments?* Cambridge: Polity.

Smart, C., Neale, B. and Wade, A. (2001) *The Changing Experience of Childhood: Families and Divorce*, Cambridge: Polity.

Social Research Association (2003) *Ethical Guidelines*, Scotland: Social Research Association. Available at <www.the-sra.org.uk/ethicals.htm> (Accessed 30 May 2013).

Spensky, M. (1992) 'Producers of legitimacy: homes for unmarried mothers in the 1950s', in C. Smart (ed) *Regulating Womanhood: Historical essays on marriage, motherhood and sexuality*, pp. 100–118, London: Routledge.

Strathern, M. (1992) *Reproducing the Future: Essays on Anthropology, Kinship and the New Reproductive Technologies,* Manchester: Manchester University Press.

Strathern, M. (1995) 'Displacing knowledge: Technology and the consequences for kinship', in F. Ginsburg and R. Rapp (eds) *Conceiving the New World Order: The Global Politics of Reproduction,* pp. 346–363 Berkeley: University of California Press.

Strathern, M. (1999) *Property, Substance and Effect: Anthropological Essays on Persons and Things,* London: Athlone Press.

Strathern, M. (2005) *Kinship, Law and the Unexpected: Relatives Are Always a Surprise,* Cambridge: Cambridge University Press.

Thompson, C. (2001) 'Strategic naturalizing: Kinship in an infertility clinic', in S. Franklin and S. McKinnon (eds) *Relative Values: Reconfiguring Kinship Studies,* pp. 175–202 Durham: Duke University Press.

Thompson, C. (2005) *Making Parents: The Ontological Choreography of Reproductive Technologies,* Cambridge, Massachusetts: MIT.

Turkmendag, I. (2012) 'The donor-conceived child's "right to personal identity": The public debate on donor anonymity in the United Kingdom', *Journal of Law and Society,* 39(1): 58–75.

Wallbank, J. (2002) 'Too many mothers? Surrogacy, kinship and the welfare of the child', *Medical Law Review* 10: 271–294.

Zerubavel, E. (2006) *The Elephant in the Room: Silence and Denial in Everyday Life,* Oxford: Oxford University Press.

Zerubavel, E. (2012) *Ancestors and Relatives: Genealogy, Identity and Community,* Oxford: Oxford University Press.

Index

Note: Locators with 'ff' refer to following folios

Adie, Kate, 23
adoption, 12–13, 17–23, 27, 31, 36,
  38, 42, 45, 60–1, 88, 93, 126,
  128, 129, 151, 158, 161
artificial insemination by donor,
  3, 20

belonging, 8, 13, 24, 26–8, 56, 66–7,
  129–34, 135, 143, 164
BioNews, 148, 149
birth mother, 14, 20, 22–3, 42, 43–5,
  60–1, 65, 66, 135, 158, 173–5
Bloklan, Talja, 25
blood, 9, 12, 13, 108, 123, 125, 127,
  128, 142–3, 145–8
  bad blood, 146–7, 148
Brown, Louise, 5, 12

Carey, Nessa, 147, 149, 155
Carsten, Janet, 24, 27, 127, 138,
  151–3, 162
connectedness, 8, 9, 10, 26, 27, 56,
  112, 113, 119–21, 125, 133,
  138–43, 145, 153, 161
court cases, 13, 16
cultural beliefs, 4, 70, 123, 156, 161

Dawkins, Richard, 148, 150
Degnen, Catherine, 154–5
disapproval, 71–2, 75, 96
discrimination, 24, 62–5
DNA, 148
donors
  anonymous, 39–43, 55, 61, 115,
    116, 174–5
  identity release, 5–6, 39, 41,
    109, 110

known, 3, 9, 39, 40–3, 46, 61, 64,
  106–7, 116–23, 124
unknown, 3, 106, 107–9, 114, 123
donor conception network, xi, 88,
  89, 92, 113, 181
donor identity, 5–6, 39, 41, 42, 80,
  83, 106, 108, 109, 110, 114–15
donor kin/kinship, 9, 106, 111,
  112–13, 118, 123
donor sibling, 106, 107, 109–12, 124

Edwards, Jeanette, 27, 70, 113,
  152–5, 159
epigenetics, 148, 155
ethic of openness, 89
ethical guidelines, 88
eugenic thinking, 155
egg donation, 5, 14, 21, 23, 32, 35,
  39, 41, 43, 57, 68, 70, 71, 72, 93,
  108, 115, 117, 126–31, 134, 152,
  158, 167, 168
embryo donation, 5, 6, 21, 56, 68,
  84, 129, 167–8, 171

Family Law Reform Act 1987, 151
family practices, 13, 26–7, 28, 120
family resemblances, 26–7, 126–7,
  132–6, 139–43, 167
family rituals, 153
family tree, 24, 56, 92
female parent, 45
fertility baby, 78, 101
financial support, 51
Finch, Janet, 27, 76, 97, 138,
  152–3, 162
future, the, 34–6, 59, 60, 69, 83–5,
  110, 112, 121, 123, 148

gametes, 3, 12, 14, 21, 36, 48, 88, 89, 106, 109, 110, 125, 131, 157, 160–1, 163, 164
genes, 4, 9, 24, 28, 30, 37, 38, 45–6, 108, 118, 125–6, 127–8, 130, 132, 134, 142, 143, 144–61, 163
bad genes, 144, 146
stranger genes, 30, 126, 127, 134, 142, 158
genetic determinism, 145, 155, 162
genetic kin/kinship, 9, 13, 27, 62, 70, 73, 118, 119, 129, 138, 144ff
genetic origins, 84, 87, 134, 135, 136, 62, 163
gestation, 36, 127, 158
Goffman, Erving, 25
grief, 33, 34, 39, 44, 46, 47, 54, 141–2
grandparents, 17, 28, 35, 49–50, 53, 56–67, 69, 73–9, 85–6, 88, 96, 99–101, 104, 107, 108, 111, 117–19, 142, 143, 150, 151, 153, 156, 161–5, 166–8

hate, 34, 91
home conception, 40, 55
Howell, Signe, 134, 153
Human Fertilisation and Embryology Act 1990, 5, 180
Human Fertilisation and Embryology Act 2008, 88, 180
Human Fertilisation and Embryology Authority, 5, 22, 110, 180, 182
human genome, 155–6

idioms, 145, 146, 159
illegitimacy/illegitimate, 18, 19, 24, 147, 151, 152
infertility, 2, 4, 5, 16, 29, 30, 32–5, 44, 46, 47, 49–53, 60, 66, 74, 79, 84, 88, 104, 141, 160
infertility clinic, 1, 3, 5, 6, 7, 13, 22, 29, 31, 35, 39–41, 43, 50, 80, 89, 106, 112, 114–17

In vitro fertilisation (IVF), 1, 4, 5, 21, 30, 31, 44, 51, 54, 74, 77, 82, 90, 91, 96, 180

Jolie, Angelina, 148
Jones, Steve, 145–7, 148, 149

Keating, Jenny, 12, 18
kinship, 10, 16–18, 27, 58, 60, 70–3, 83, 85, 107, 111–14, 117, 118, 119, 123–4, 127–31, 138, 143, 144ff
de-kinning, 20, 153
kinning, 153
Konrad, Monica, 23, 36, 109, 110, 111, 113, 127

Lawler, Steph, 24
Lewis, Jane, 12, 20
lineage, 24, 48, 142, 159
Local Government Act 1988, 181
love, 28, 57, 62, 82, 99, 104, 120, 131–2, 138, 154, 159
'over-loved', 58–9

manhood, 32–4
Martin, Emily, 149–50
Mason, Jennifer, xi, 27, 76, 97, 108, 131, 132, 138, 153, 162, 167
May, Vanessa, xi, 26
metaphor, 108, 147, 148–50, 156, 157, 158
Midgley, Mary, 150
Morgan, David, 12, 26, 120, 131

narrative(s), 8, 11, 13, 24–5, 57, 60, 88–9, 92, 103, 130, 145, 157–8, 162, 165
nature, 12, 128, 146, 150, 154–5, 159, 160
non-genetic grandparents, 61, 138, 142
Nurse, Sir Paul, 181
nurture, 127, 128, 132, 150, 152, 154–5, 163

openness, 8, 21, 71, 72, 76, 87ff,
171, 181

paternity, 14, 39, 84, 151, 152
personal identity, 13, 23–6,
70–1, 137
popular/public imagination, 4, 12,
24, 146, 147, 149
pregnancy/pregnant, 3, 19, 29, 30,
33, 34, 36–7, 40, 43, 44, 46, 48,
49ff, 78, 84, 96, 112,
121, 126ff
privacy, 55, 70–1, 83, 86,
103–4
private lives, 12, 102, 104

relatedness, 16, 27, 107, 117–21,
125, 132, 136, 145, 150–5,
157, 161
relationality, 90, 113, 124

rights
of child, 42, 80, 87, 89, 106
of parents, 14, 16, 18, 45
of sperm donor, 13, 42
to privacy, 70–1, 83
Rose, Steven, 147, 148–9, 155

Sales, Sally, 12, 18, 20, 93
secrecy, 8, 13, 68, 76, 82, 83, 88
social practices, 6, 19, 108, 124,
129–32, 156
Strathern, Marilyn, 70, 73, 83, 113,
127, 128, 131, 134

The Times, 11
The Guardian, 11
transilient relationship, 111–12
Turkmendag, Ilke, 22, 23, 88

womanhood, 7, 30, 35–6, 126

Printed and bound in Great Britain by
CPI Group (UK) Ltd, Croydon, CR0 4YY